Color Atlas of Orofacial Diseases

Second Edition

W. R. Tyldesley

D.D.S., Ph.D., M.Sc., F.D.S.R.C.S.
Former Dean of Dental Studies
University of Liverpool
England

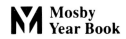

Mosby
Year Book

St. Louis   Baltimore   Boston   Chicago   London   Philadelphia   Sydney   Toronto

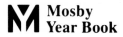

**Mosby
Year Book**

Dedicated to Publishing Excellence

Mosby–Year Book, Inc.
11830 Westline Drive
St. Louis, MO 63146

Copyright © 1991 Second Edition W.R. Tyldesley
All rights reserved.
Published with rights in the USA, Canada and Puerto Rico by
Mosby–Year Book, Inc.

ISBN 0-8016-6293-1

English second edition first published in 1991 by Wolfe Publishing
Ltd, 2–16 Torrington Place, London WC1E 7LT, UK.

First edition 1971 by L.W. Kay and R. Haskell

Printed in the Netherlands.

**Library of Congress Cataloging-in-Publication Data has been
applied for.**

Contents

Preface

The first edition of this atlas was published in 1971. Since then it has had a worldwide distribution and has become a standard aid in the study of diseases of the orofacial region by practitioners of both medicine and dentistry. The introduction to the first edition included the hope that it would be of value to students (both undergraduate and postgraduate) and also to established members of the professions as an *aide-mémoire* and refresher course. This hope seems to have been fully realized.

After almost 20 years it was thought desirable to produce a new and updated edition of the *Atlas*. Following the sad death of Lester Kay, Dr. Haskell felt that he did not wish to embark on the production of the second edition, and gave his blessing to the present author. Although, as is described below, the main outline remains as it was in the first edition, many of the illustrations have been replaced. It is quite evident that in these circumstances archival material and that supplied by colleagues must be used. This means that uniformity in such matters as colour balance is impossible to attain: in the author's *Colour Atlas of Oral Medicine*, most of the illustrations are from photographs taken by the author under uniform conditions. This is, quite clearly, not the case in the present compilation.

Of the 394 illustrations, 261 are new to this edition. Most of these have been taken by the present author or are a part of the collection started, at the School of Dentistry of the University of Liverpool, by Prof. E.D. Farmer. There is a substantial contribution by two colleagues from the Maxillofacial Surgery Unit at Walton Hospital, Liverpool. Mr E.D. Vaughan has allowed the use of illustrations of a number of his patients with neoplastic and associated lesions, some of them very unusual; while Mr. O.A. Pospisil has contributed material for the last section of the *Atlas*, showing a wide spectrum of clinical presentations of developmental abnormalities of the jaws. Miss E.M. Theil has provided slides of a range of periodontal conditions, and Mr. A. Milosevic has also contributed. The illustrations of the oral manifestations of AIDS are reprinted from *A Colour Atlas of AIDS* by kind permission of Dr. C.E. Farthing and his colleagues. If any loaned illustrations remain from those acknowledged in the first edition, the current author must present his apologies to the original owners.

The arrangement of the material in this edition is based, as was that in the first edition, on both the clinical and anatomical features of the conditions. The sections have been arranged to bring together lesions of similar appearance (as in "Facial swellings") or of the same site (as in "The tongue"). This clinical approach to the problem was adopted in the full knowledge that some inconsistencies might arise. Nonetheless, it is felt by the present author, as it was by the original authors, that this is by far the most practical approach. The sectional divisions are not entirely rigid: a number of conditions appear more than once, in different sections, in order to maintain completeness within the sections. As far as possible there is continuity between the sections—although this has not been possible to attain in every case.

It goes without saying that the original authors' warning still stands: "Although a guide to intelligent diagnosis, a book of this type must never be regarded as a substitute for the detailed practical study of actual cases".

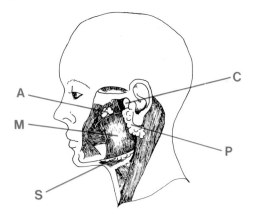

1 The relationship between the masseter muscle (M), the head of the mandibular condyle (C), the parotid gland (P), the accessory parotid (A) and the submandibular gland (S). These structures are frequently confused on clinical examination.

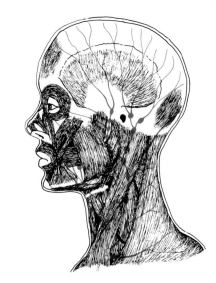

2 The usual distribution of the lymph nodes associated with the oral and facial tissues.

Facial swellings

By far the most common cause of facial swelling is dental infection. However, there are many other possibilities to be considered. The clinical details and, particularly, the anatomical features involved must be taken into account when making an initial diagnosis. An example of the importance of the anatomical approach to diagnosis is that of masseteric swelling, which very frequently is confused initially with parotid swelling. Bony changes, inflammatory, metabolic or neoplastic, may also simulate and be confused with simple soft-tissue swellings. Salivary gland swellings may easily be confused with those of closely associated lymph nodes or of other soft tissue structures.

Although the figures in this section represent the most characteristic features of the conditions described, it must again be stressed that a full clinical examination is essential for an accurate diagnosis.

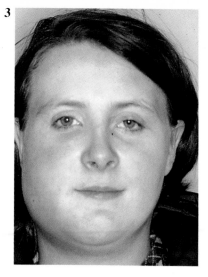

3,4 Dental infection The most common cause of facial swelling is infection of dental origin. This is usually the result of a periapical dentoalveolar abscess, which spreads into the facial tissues following perforation of the alveolar bone by pus. The clinical characteristics are, therefore, initial severe pain during the intrabony phase, followed by a sudden relief of pain on perforation of the bone and the release of pressure. Oedema of the soft tissues follows (**3**), and then increasing pain with the spread of the infective process (**4**).

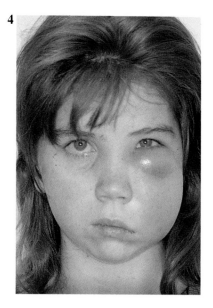

5 Infected antrum Other intra-bony sources of infection — such as infected cysts, for example — may result in facial swelling if there is spread of the infective process to the soft tissues. **5** is a very unusual example of such a spreading infection following packing of the maxillary sinus. Clearly, in circumstances such as these the clinical pattern will not follow that outlined above (**3,4**).

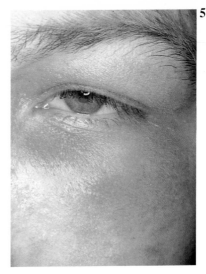

6 Facial sinus If the infection localizes, either spontaneously or as a result of antibiotic treatment, external pointing may occur and, eventually, an external sinus may be established. **6** shows the imminent establishment of a facial sinus in an inadequately treated infection following a dental abscess.

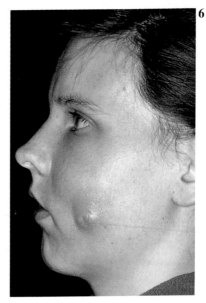

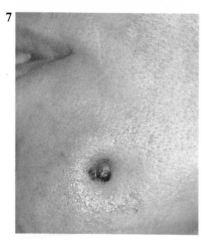

7 Facial sinus This is an established facial sinus originating from an area of chronic apical infection on a lower anterior tooth. These lesions are often misdiagnosed in the absence of any obvious source of infection — a basal cell carcinoma is often suspected. A mistaken diagnosis is particularly likely if the patient is apparently edentulous, but has (for instance) an unsuspected retained root as the source of infection.

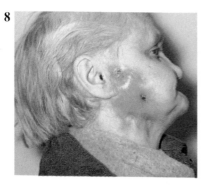

8 Facial sinus Very occasionally more extensive, possibly multiple, facial sinuses may result from intrabony infected lesions that have been difficult to treat surgically or involve organisms that present problems of antibiotic resistance. The facial lesion in **8** is the result of secondary infection of a keratocyst of the mandible by organisms that presented difficult problems of antibiotic treatment in this patient, who had multiple adverse drug reactions.

9,10 Actinomycosis Not all soft tissue infections of the facial regions result from the spread of dental or intrabony infections, although most do so. **9** illustrates the classic condition of cervico-facial actinomycosis: probably an opportunistic infection following some form of trauma (which might, for instance, be a dental extraction). The *Actinomyces* species are normally commensal in the mouth and pharynx. The involvement of the skin is quite characteristic; considerable scarring may remain after treatment.

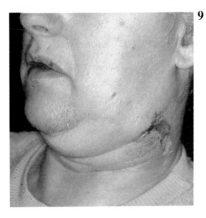

10 shows the characteristic pus obtained from this lesion, containing the so called "sulphur granules". These are discrete aggregates of the filaments of the organism.

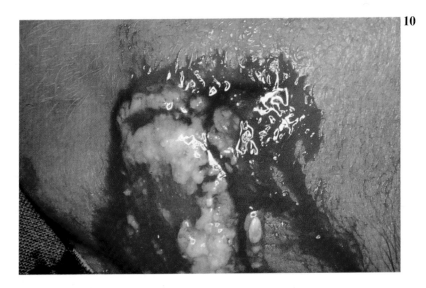

11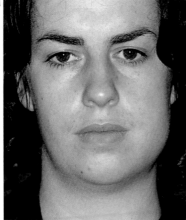

11,12 Lymphoma In a few instances it may be difficult to distinguish between infective lesions of dental origin involving the soft tissues of the face and primary soft tissue lesions involving the facial bones. In **11** is shown a lymphoma in the facial soft tissues that was at first thought to be a lesion of dental origin. The radiograph (**12**), although in retrospect not clearly indicating a periodontal condition, initially was interpreted as doing so. It eventually became clear that the bone loss associated with the teeth represented infiltration of the periodontium by the neoplastic tissue.

12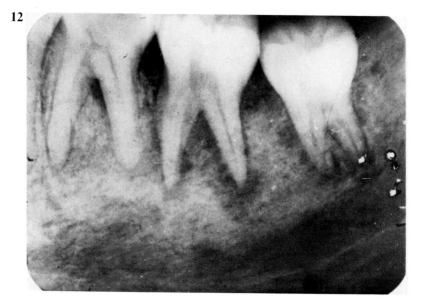

13,14 Myxosarcoma A situation the reverse of that illustrated in **11** and **12** is shown. In this case a myxosarcoma arising in the maxilla (**13**) has spread directly into the soft tissues of the face. As in the previous case, it was initially diagnosed as a dental problem: the first sign of the neoplasm was a mobile and tender maxillary first molar. A dental abscess was thought to be responsible.

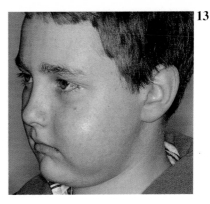

13

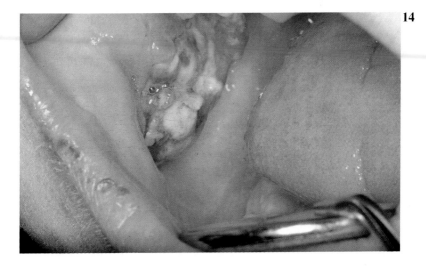

14

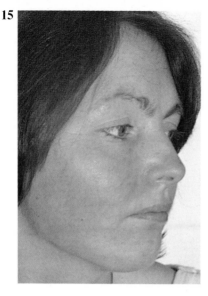

15,16 Angio-oedema Soft tissue facial swelling, particularly of the lip, is common in angio-oedema or in allergic oedema. Again, lack of appreciation of the clinical features may result in an initial incorrect diagnosis of dental infection. The patient shown in **15** is known to have hereditary angio-oedema. **16** shows a relatively mild (and therefore easily mistaken) allergic reaction to penicillin.

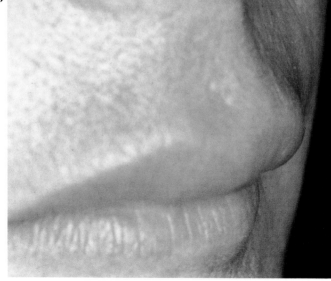

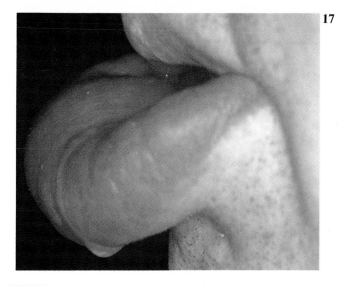

17 Crohn's disease Facial swelling, which may become gross and may particularly affect the lips, may be a prominent feature of oral Crohn's disease or of the closely related orofacial granulomatosis. This patient, with established lower gut Crohn's disease, shows the most common marker of oral Crohn's disease: a swollen lower lip; in this case, grossly so. He also has proliferative buccal lesions containing characteristic non caseating tuberculoid granulomas and prominent palpable cervical lymph nodes. It is believed that the cause of the facial swelling is local lymph node obstruction — a situation similar to that in Crohn's disease, which affects other sites in the gastrointestinal tract. There is currently much interest in the suggested association of this group of conditions with food allergy. (See also **174, 175**.)

18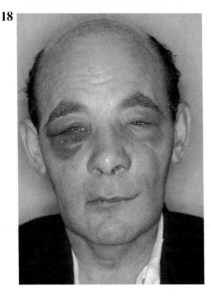

18 Anticoagulant therapy
Bleeding into the soft tissues of the face of a patient on inadequately controlled anticoagulant therapy has caused facial swelling. At first sight this resembles a simple black eye, although there is no history of trauma. Since it is not a particularly painful process, and since there is evident bruising, an alternative diagnosis of a dental infection should not complicate the issue. A similar situation may occur in haematological diseases in which the coagulation mechanism is deficient. In leukaemias, for instance, there may be a thrombocytopenia.

19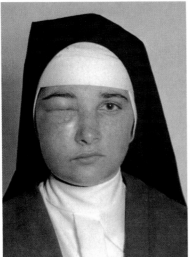

19 Surgical emphysema This is surgical emphysema: air has been introduced into the facial soft tissues by the use of compressed air during dental treatment. It may also occur as a result of facial trauma, usually involving a fracture of the antral walls. The condition is of sudden onset and, although it superficially resembles the result of acute infection, it is painless and the history is entirely different. The classic sign is of crepitus (a crackling sensation when pressing on the tissues), although this is sometimes difficult to demonstrate.

20 Salivary calculus Swelling of the submandibular salivary gland due to duct obstruction by a calculus is shown here. In these circumstances the degree of swelling and discomfort is often directly associated with meals, the increased salivary flow induced by food causing an increase in back pressure in the gland. In long standing cases degenerative and inflammatory changes in the gland may lead to permanent swelling.

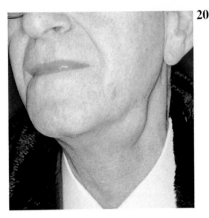

20

21 Submandibular duct obstruction Secondary bacterial infection of the gland, either acute or chronic sialadenitis, may also occur following obstruction of the submandibular duct. Acute infections of this kind are often very painful. In this case repeated obstructive episodes have been followed by an acute infection. The differential diagnosis between this situation and the involvement of submandibular lymph nodes in an acute dental infection is an important one that depends on careful clinical assessment and, in particular, the past history.

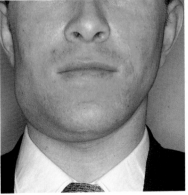

21

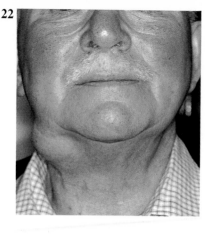

22 Neoplasms of the salivary glands Neoplasms of the salivary glands probably represent about 3% of all tumours on a worldwide basis, although this figure is only one in the range of from 0.1% to 5% quoted by different authorities and varying according to the precise criteria adopted. Of tumours of the major glands about 90% are of the parotid and about 10% of the submandibular gland. Sublingual gland tumours are rare. Shown here is the slowly growing, firm, painless swelling of the submandibular gland that is characteristic of a neoplasm arising in the gland. The most common neoplasm in this site is some form of adenoma, a pleomorphic adenoma being the most likely. Although the growth of the neoplasm may in itself be pain free, obstruction of salivary flow may occur, leading to symptoms outlined above (**20,21**). It is evident that careful clinical investigation, possibly including the use of contrast radiography and imaging techniques, will be needed fully to assess the situation.

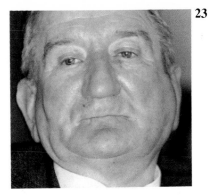

23,24 Parotid swelling The parotid glands may undergo obstructive, degenerative and inflammatory changes similar to those described in the submandibular glands (**21,22**). More often these changes are bilateral and associated with the generalized changes of Sjögren's syndrome or related conditions. Frequently the complex of degenerative and inflammatory changes is difficult fully to elucidate. Calcification may occur in the gland substance following on long-term changes of this kind. **23** shows a patient with such long-term changes in the parotid glands, with frequent episodes of acute infection superimposed on the chronic degenerative condition. Intraorally, the parotid duct papillae may be inflamed and swollen (**24**).

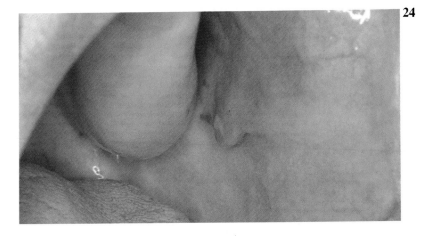

25

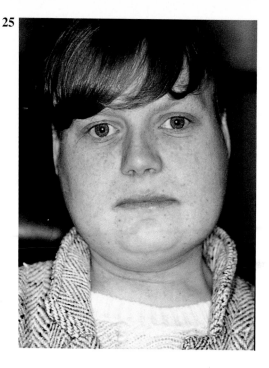

25 Mumps Acute and chronic bacterial infections of the parotid glands may occur just as in the case of the submandibular glands (**21**). However, the most common infection of the parotid glands, mumps, is viral in origin. Although the condition is generally bilateral, one parotid gland is often particularly affected; the submandibular glands may also be involved. Affected glands are tender and painful. The patient feels ill, and there is a general malaise and fever. Mumps often occurs in minor epidemics. The young female patient in **25** has mumps for the second time: a very unusual situation, since the immune system normally protects against a second attack by the virus.

26,27 Pleomorphic adenomas of the parotid glands Neoplasms in the parotid gland constitute 90% of all salivary gland tumours. Of these, 65% are pleomorphic adenomas. **26** shows the typical presentation of such a pleomorphic adenoma of the body of the parotid. However, it should always be remembered that the accessory parotid tissue may be involved in any kind of salivary gland changes. **27** shows an adenoma originating in the accessory parotid.

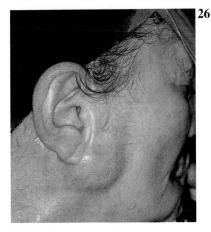

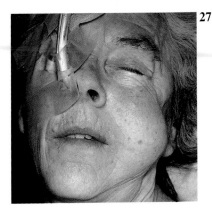

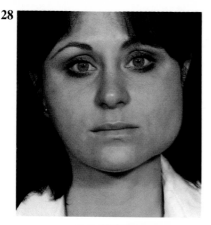

28 Masseteric hypertrophy Perhaps the most common misdiagnosis of parotid swelling involves failure to recognise masseteric hypertrophy. This is a not uncommon condition, although the cause is unknown; occlusal problems have been suggested, but there is little evidence for this. The anatomical definition of the masseter muscle is generally all that is necessary to differentiate this condition from parotid swelling. Occasionally this condition may occur bilaterally.

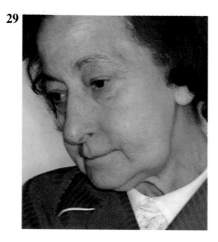

29 Cervical nodes The involvement of cervical lymph nodes in dental infections has been mentioned above (**21**). However, a very significant source of cervical lymph node abnormality occurs in neoplastic processes. The existence, or otherwise, of cervical nodes containing malignant cells is a vital indicator of the prognosis of an oral carcinoma. **29** shows well developed visible and palpable cervical nodes in a patient with advanced carcinoma of the floor of the mouth.

30 Cervical nodes Shown are the rather less well defined bilateral cervical nodes in a patient with Hodgkin's lymphoma. The cervical lymph nodes are the most common site in the head and neck for the presentation of lymphomas of all types, although extra nodal lesions may occur (as in **11,12**).

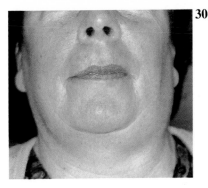

31 Neoplastic bony changes Evidently, neoplastic bony changes will lead to a change in facial contour. Even the most superficial of examinations would show that this facial distortion, the result of a myxofibroma of the maxilla, was of skeletal origin. The changes resulting from distortion of the orbital walls are evident.

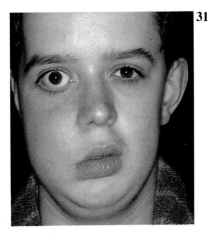

32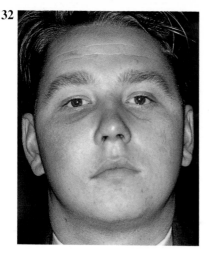

32,33,34,35 Changes in facial contour Changes in the contour of the facial skeleton may mistakenly be thought, on superficial viewing, to be of soft tissue origin. **32** shows the altered facial contour of a patient with monostotic fibrous dysplasia of the right maxilla. Changes in facial contour are often best appreciated by taking a view such as that shown in **33** (or the opposite view from the top of the head downwards). Intraoral examination (**34**) and suitable radiographs (**35**) are, evidently,

33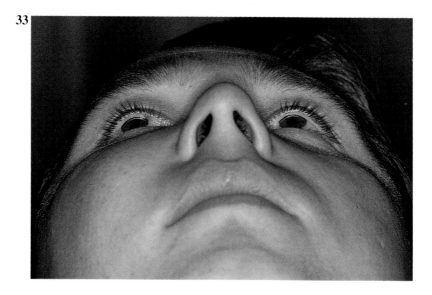

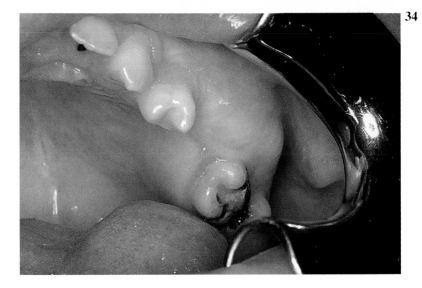

essential to even a preliminary diagnosis. The definitive diagnosis of monostotic fibrous dysplasia is by biopsy: there are no characteristic biochemical changes. Monostotic fibrous dysplasia affects only a single segment of the jaws, with no other skeletal involvement. In other parts of the skeleton it may affect other single bones.

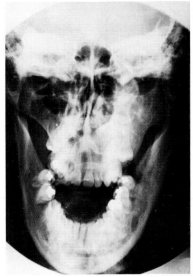

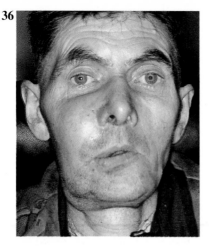

36,37 Carcinoma of the antrum
Facial distortion may also occur as a result of maxillary expansion due to carcinoma of the antrum (**36**). Just as in the case of the entirely benign fibrous dysplasia, intraoral and radiographic changes are likely to be detectable by the time significant facial abnormality is seen (**37**).

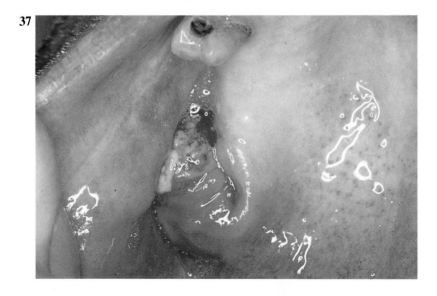

38,39 Carcinoma of the antrum
In this patient an antral carcinoma has destroyed the wall of the maxilla and is involving the facial tissues by local spread. Intra-orally (**39**) there is expansion of the maxilla with early soft tissue involvement, much as is shown in **37**.

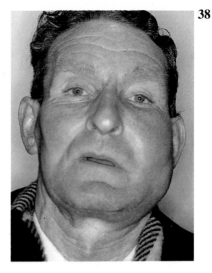

38

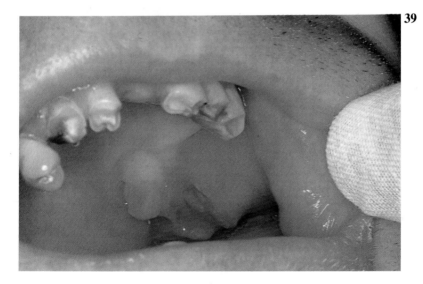

39

40

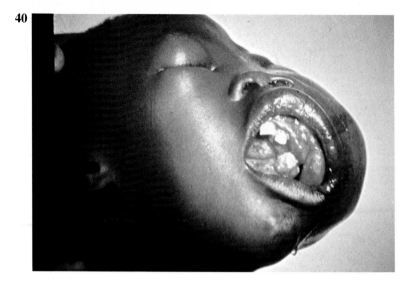

40 Burkitt's lymphoma Burkitt's lymphoma, the malignant disease of childhood endemic to parts of tropical Africa, characteristically affects the jaws and, particularly, the maxilla, as in this case.

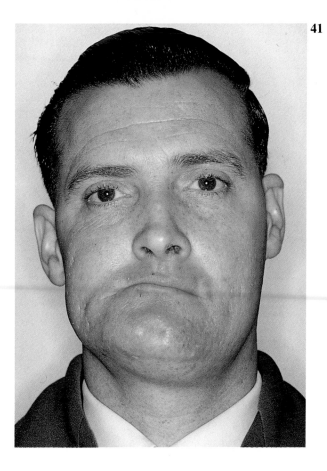

41 Condylar hyperplasia Mandibular distortion may also occur, as a result of either simple or neoplastic changes. The gross distortion of the mandible in **41** is due to a simple hyperplasia of one condyle head. The condition apparently represents a continuation or reactivation of the condylar growth centres, which normally cease to function at around the age of 20 years.

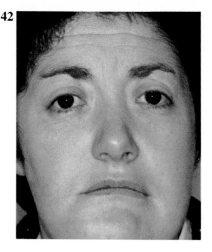

42,43 Expansion of intrabony carcinoma A facial distortion quite similar to the one shown in **41** may occur as a result of neoplastic or cystic growth in the mandible. This mandibular asymmetry resulted from the expansion of an intrabony carcinoma — a very rare lesion as a primary neoplasm.

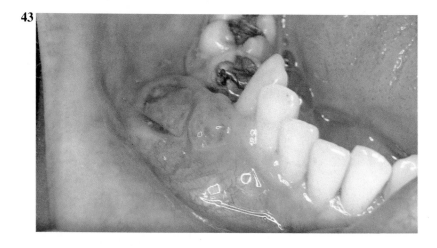

44 Unilateral condylar hypoplasia Mandibular asymmetry may also result from damage to a condylar growth centre during childhood, leading to unilateral condylar hypoplasia and lack of mandibular development: in this case as a result of a severe middle ear infection.

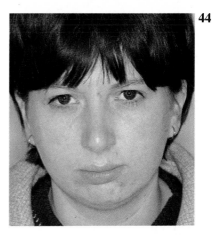

45 Branchial cyst A branchial cyst, situated superficially in the soft tissues of the neck, below the angle of the mandible and anterior to the sternomastoid muscle. These cysts may become very large, and are thought to develop from epithelial remnants of embryonic clefts. They may occur at any age and are, in general, symptom free. They may be mistaken for enlarged cervical lymph nodes, although the fluid contents give a quite different texture on palpation.

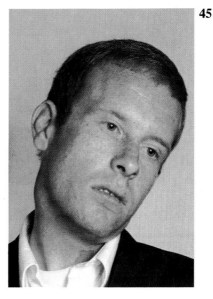

46

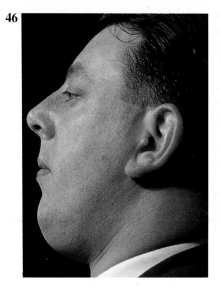

46 Dermoid cyst This is a dermoid cyst occurring in the floor of the mouth but expanding visibly below the level of the mandible. Such cysts, as in this case, are often in the mid line, although laterally placed cysts may occur. There is some controversy as to whether they originate solely above the mylo-hyoid muscle or, in some cases, below it. These cysts are also considered to arise from embryonic remnants, but in contrast to branchial cysts the walls may contain dermal structures such as hair follicles or sweat glands.

Lips and facial skin

The lips and the surrounding skin behave in a rather idiosyncratic manner, often reacting partly as mucous membrane and partly as skin. Some lesions, such as those of facial herpes, have a strong predilection for the mucosal–skin junction of the lips. Many lesions affecting the perioral area depend on the local anatomy, which is paralleled only in the ano-genital skin — mucous membrane junction. For example, angular cheilitis has some similarities to anal fissuers; and both may occur in Crohn's disease.

The facial skin in general is susceptible to all forms of skin disease. However, some diseases are far more likely to appear on the facial skin (often in characteristic form) than are others, and these have been shown in this section. The exposure of the facial skin to sunlight may play a significant part in the production of some lesions (such as actinic cheilitis) or in their severity (as in chronic discoid lupus).

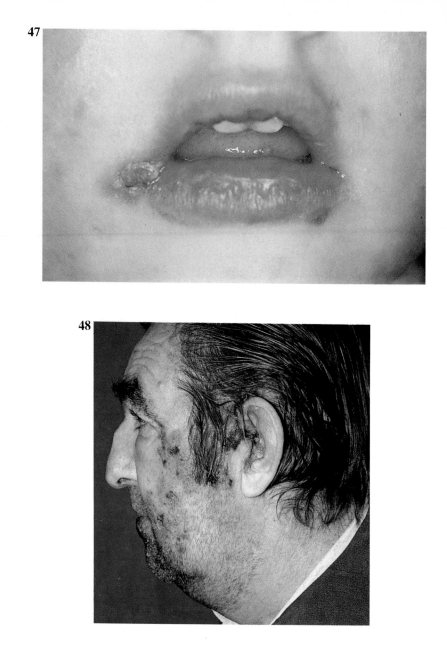

47,48,49 Primary herpetic stomatitis Primary herpes simplex most commonly appears as a predominantly oral mucosal condition: primary herpetic stomatitis (**49**). The lesions of the facial skin may vary from a few perioral vesicles (**47**) to much more extensive areas of multiple vesicle formation (**48**). The unilateral distribution of the lesions shown in **48** and **49** is to some extent similar to that usually seen in herpes zoster. However, the skin lesions in this patient are not confined to the distribution of one branch of the trigeminal distribution, as is usual in herpes zoster (**53**). In general there is less actual pain, as distinct from irritation, than in herpes zoster. In doubtful cases only virological and antibody studies can distinguish the two. There is no clinical difference between herpes simplex type 1 and type 2 infections. Widespread and intractable herpes simplex infections may occur in drug induced immunosuppression (as in transplant patients), and persistent herpes may be one of the markers of AIDS.

49

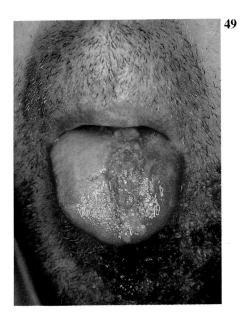

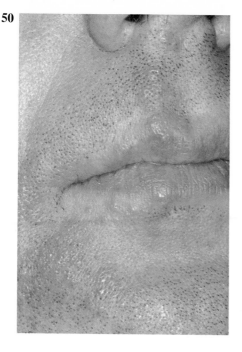

50,51,52 Recurrent herpes
Following an episode of primary herpes simplex infection, approximately half of those patients with an intact immune system develop longterm recurrent lesions that mainly affect the perioral skin. Following the early vesicular phase and prevesicular erythema (**50**), the vesicles break down to form the familiar crusted lesions (**51**). In patients with immunodeficiencies these lesions may be much more widespread. **52** shows more widespread herpetic lesions of the chin in a patient with chronic lymphocytic leukaemia.

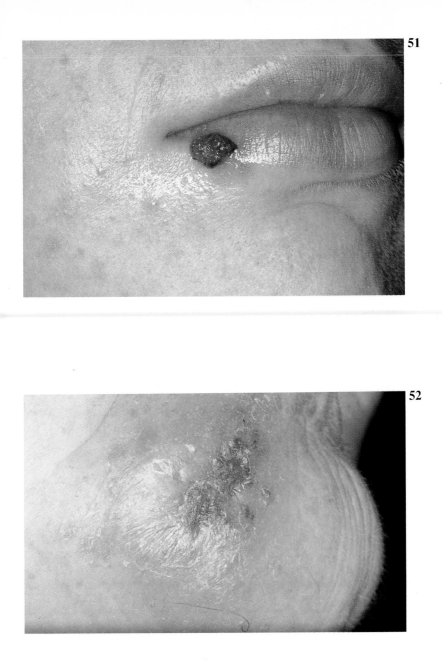

53

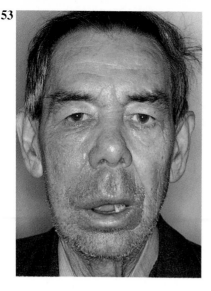

54

53,54 Herpes zoster In the early stages of herpes zoster, pain in the affected area may be severe. This may occur before the development of vesicles. The distribution of the vesicles in the area of the ophthalmic division of the trigeminal nerve (**53**) is the most common, although more than one division may occasionally be involved, as may cervical nerves. The rash is very variable; it may be relatively diffuse, and the vesicles may appear over a period of some days. In other cases the vesicles appear simultaneously and densely packed. There may be secondary infection with pustule formation. Scarring of neural tissue and of facial skin may occur following resolution of the rash, and an intractable neuralgia may follow. **54** shows thickening of the facial skin and facial nerve weakness following herpes zoster affecting the right ear: the Ramsay Hunt syndrome. There is increasing evidence that vigorous early treatment with antiviral agents significantly reduces the incidence of these long-term problems.

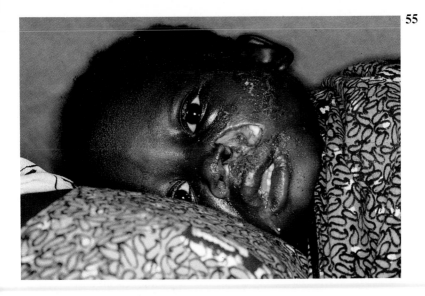

55 Cancrum oris The destructive facial lesions of cancrum oris occur as a result of the rapid spread of acute ulcerative gingivitis in young patients with an immune system impaired by malnutrition and suppressed by a viral illness (usually measles). Very occasionally similar lesions may occur in adult patients grossly debilitated by other disease processes such as acute leukaemias.

56,57 Perioral bacterial lesions Infections of the perioral skin that may resemble herpetic lesions but may be either entirely bacterial or of mixed viral-bacterial origin may occur in immunocompromised patients. **56** shows a patient with Crohn's disease taking relatively high doses of systemic steroids, but within conventional limits of therapy. The lesion shown is bacterial in origin: in this case, staphylococcal. Almost any organism may be involved (even those normally considered non pathogenic), and identification is essential for successful treatment. **57** shows another lesion of this kind in a patient with acute lymphocytic leukaemia.

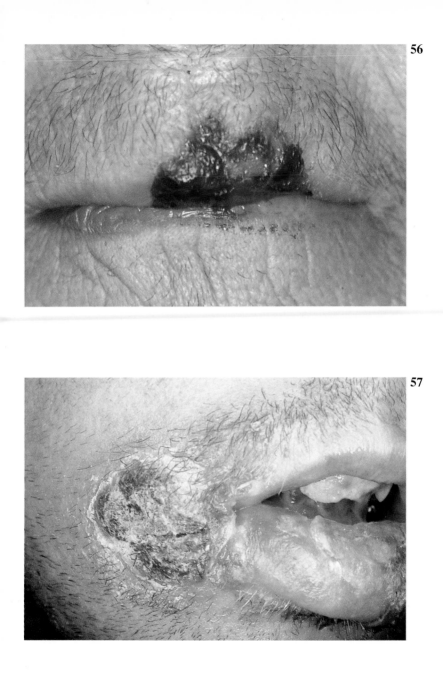

58 Angular cheilitis Angular cheilitis is a marker of some form of local or systemic abnormality. In most cases the abnormality is simply the presence of deep folds at the angle of the mouth that may be anatomical or may be the result of wearing dentures with insufficient height. The tissues become moistened with saliva and a suitable environment for the proliferation of organisms is created. In most cases the infection is by *Candida* species, in others by bacteria — usually staphylococci. In those patients with denture problems, there is often an associated oral chronic atrophic candidiasis (the so called denture stomatitis). In other cases there is an associated candidal leukoplakia of the nearby buccal mucosa. In some patients the condition may be an early indication of generalized debility, particularly as a result of haematological disease or diabetes mellitus. The patient in **58** had previously undiagnosed pernicious anaemia.

59 Commissural leukoplakia In this patient long neglect, probably combined with a heavy smoking habit, has resulted in malignant transformation of a commissural leukoplakia. The origin of the condition as an angular cheilitis is still evident.

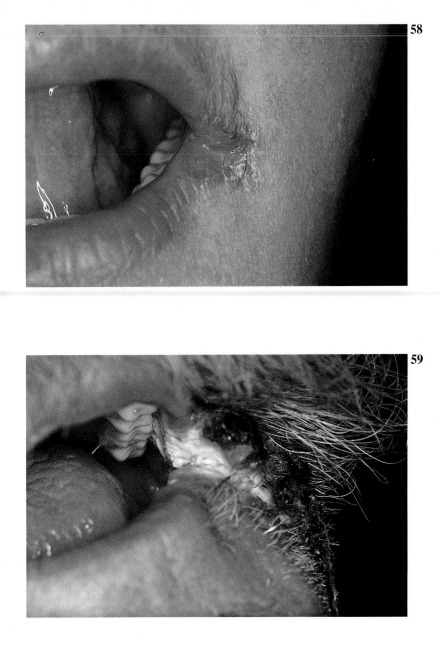

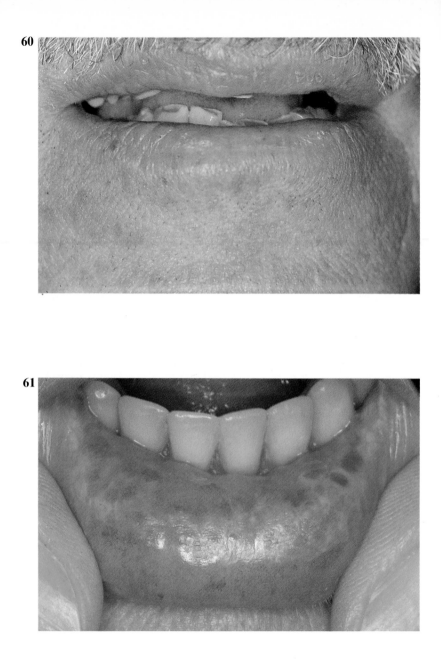

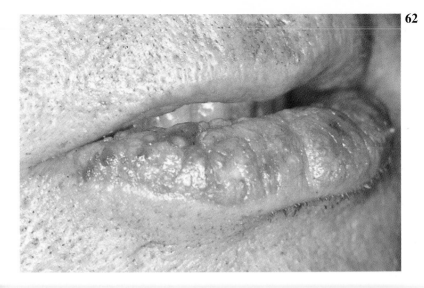

60,61,62,63 Keratoses of the lower lip Simple keratotic lesions of the lower lip such as that shown in **60** may have the histology of an entirely benign simple hyperkeratosis. There is a similar clinical appearance in some patients with lichen planus (**61**). However, in other patients, particularly those with a history of prolonged exposure to strong sunlight, a much more histologically aggressive lesion may be present. There is often crusting and induration of the lip due to a reactive fibrosis of the underlying tissues (**62**). This condition is often described as actinic cheilitis, although similar changes can occur without the background of solar exposure. It is much more common in the lower lip and in male patients. Because of its tendency to undergo

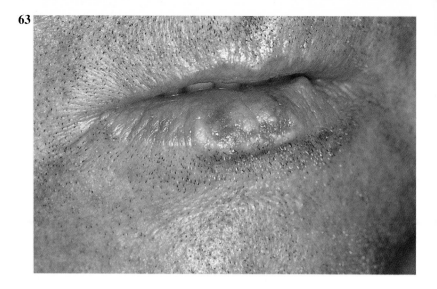

transformation into active carcinoma, as in **63**, the term lip at risk is often used.

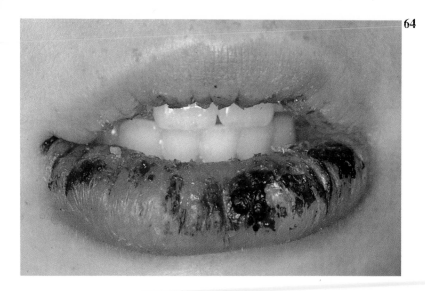

64 Exfoliative cheilitis Exfoliative cheilitis is not well understood. Occurring most frequently in young patients, there is cyclic hyperparakeratosis of the vermilion borders of the lips. Fissuring and secondary infection, usually with *Staph. aureus*, follows. There is no known association with other conditions, but stress is often reported by the patients to be a significant precipitating factor.

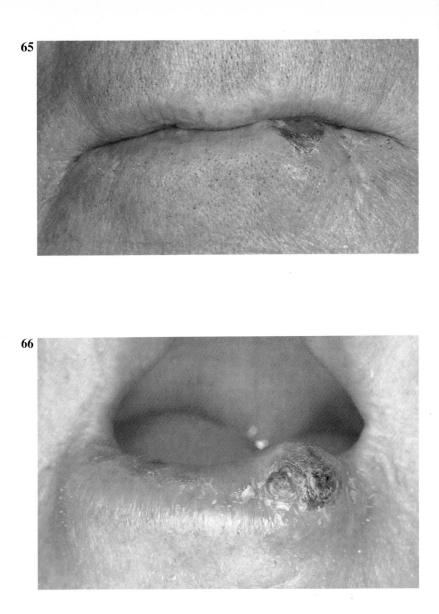

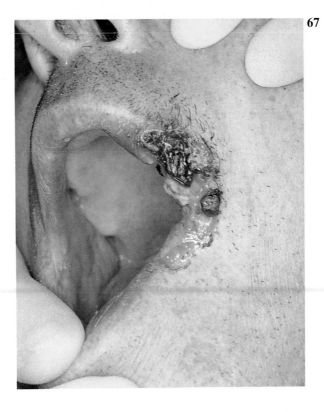

65,66,67 Carcinoma of the lip In most cases squamous cell carcinoma of the lip arises without any history of a prolonged premalignant keratosis as described in **62,63**. The lesions are predominantly of the lower lip and occur, in a high proportion of cases, in older male patients. The onset of the neoplasm and its subsequent progression are usually slow and symptomless; the lesion is often thought by the patient to be one of herpes (**65**). A considerable time may elapse before suspicions are aroused by continuing extension of the lesion (**66**). Distant spread is slow and late; relatively minor surgery is often curative. Carcinoma of the upper lip (**67**) is relatively rare, and most commonly occurs as an extension of an angular lesion, as in this case.

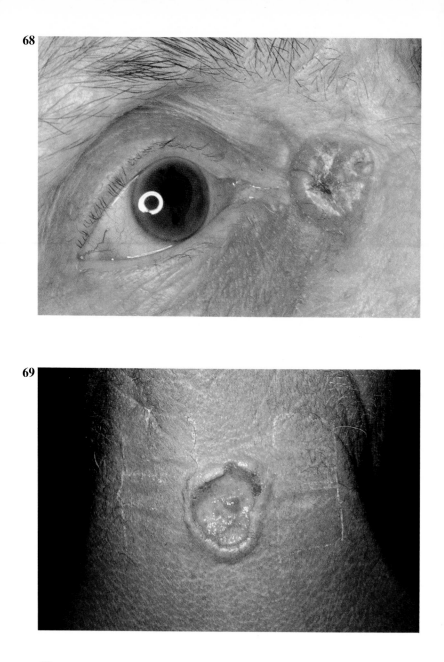

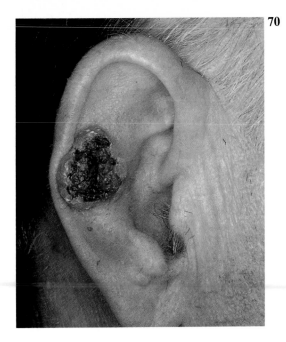

68,69,70,71,72 Basal cell carcinoma The most common neoplasm of the facial skin is the basal cell carcinoma. Although it may arise in any site, the usual location is in the upper part of the face, lateral to the nose and below the eye (**68**). The characteristic appearance is of a slowly growing ulcerated lesion with a rolled edge; a classically formed lesion of the neck is shown in **69**, and one of the ear in **70**. When the lesion is small (**71**) it can resemble an externally discharging sinus of dental origin (**72**), and there is often diagnostic confusion. A similar sinus is shown in **7**. The basal cell carcinoma virtually never produces metastases, but local growth may continue until widespread tissue destruction has taken place.

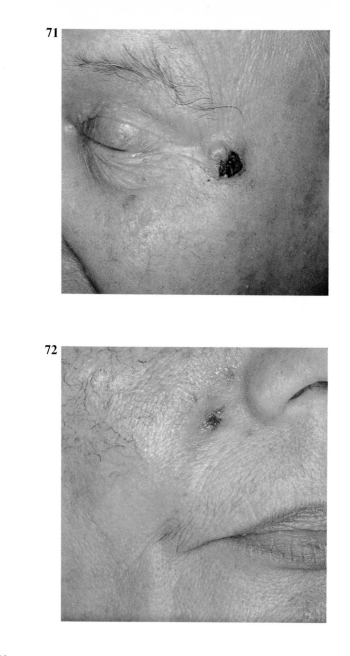

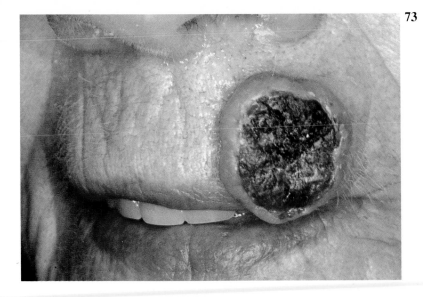

73 Kerato-acanthoma The lesion shown is a kerato-acanthoma; it predominantly occurs on the facial skin and grows rapidly. After a static period it may then regress slowly, leaving a scar. Histologically it is a hyperplastic epithelial lesion with changes verging on those seen in carcinoma. Clinically and histologically, this is a lesion that may cause great problems of diagnosis.

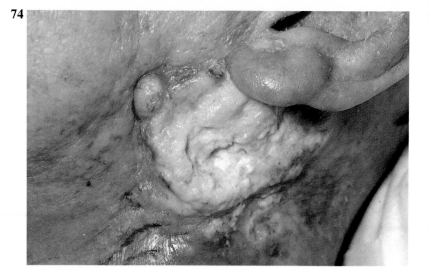

74 Squamous cell carcinoma of parotid gland   This is a squamous
cell carcinoma of the parotid gland penetrating the overlying skin.

75 Squamous cell carcinoma of external ear This squamous cell carcinoma of the external ear is a very rare lesion. Squamous cell carcinoma of the facial skin occurs much less frequently than does basal cell carcinoma.

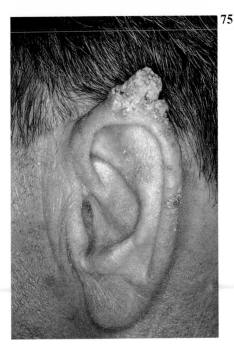

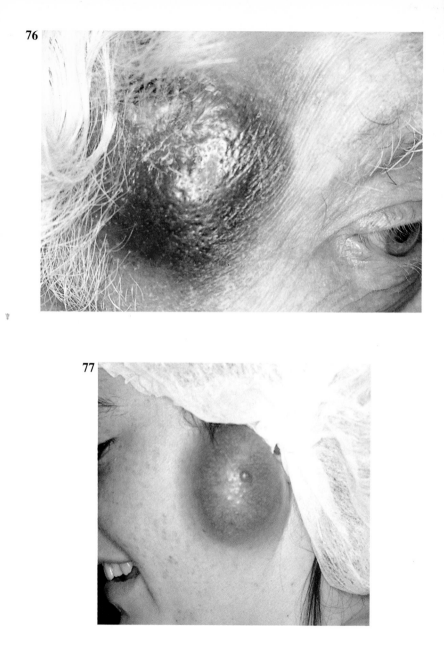

76,77,78 Neoplastic lesions of the face A wide range of neoplastic lesions may occur on the face. The definitive diagnosis of these depends on the histological findings rather than on appearance. The melanoma (**76**) is fairly characteristic in its colouring, but is not a great deal different, at least on superficial examination, from the haemangio-sarcoma shown in **77**.

Diffuse "medical" neoplasms may also present as skin deposits in the face. The patient in **78** has acute myeloid leukaemia, and the small lesions in the facial skin are deposits of malignant cells.

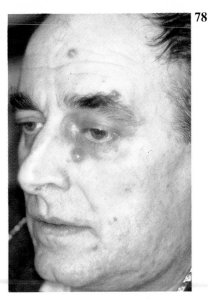

78

79 "Lick eczema" Shown here is the so called lick eczema. It is not, in fact, eczema in any form: it is the result of a lip licking habit so extensive as to involve the perioral skin. When the patient (invariably a child) can be persuaded to stop the habit, the lesion disappears at once.

80 Melanotic macules of the lips These melanotic macules of the lips are associated with intestinal polyps in the classical presentation of the Peutz–Jeghers syndrome. There may be associated similar macules distributed across the bridge of the nose. The intestinal polyps are generally benign, but occasional malignant transformation may occur. There is a genetic basis to this syndrome — it is transmitted as an autosomal dominant characteristic.

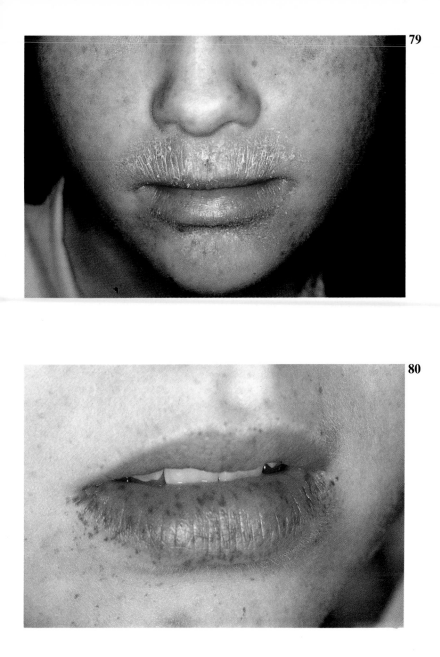

81 Traumatic lesions of the lower lip This traumatic lesion of the lower lip would be difficult to diagnose without the history. However, the maxillary left central incisor has been lost as a consequence of the same incident, and the origin of the lip lesion is obvious.

82 Electrical burn lesion of the lower lip The lower lip is particularly susceptible to trauma during the course of surgery in and around the mouth. These lesions are the result of accidental contact with an electrocautery instrument.

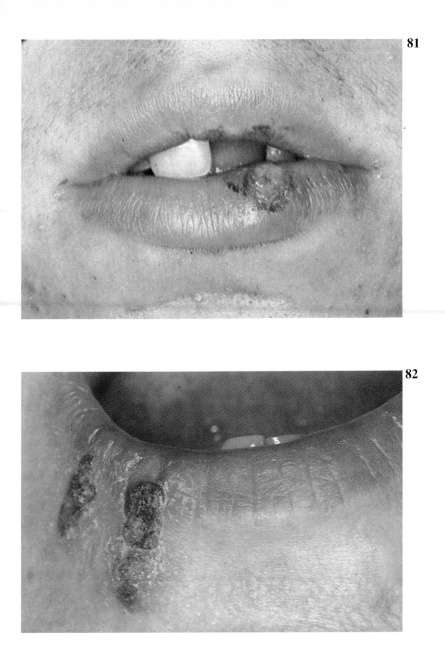

83 Rosacea This patient has rosacea, an inflammatory disease affecting the facial skin with involvement of the sebaceous glands and occasional pustule formation. A very similar condition restricted to the perioral skin is known as perioral dermatitis. The patients with this form of the condition are almost all young females.

84 Facial eczema Occasionally patients, such as this one, present with endogenous eczema restricted to the facial skin. Two sites are most often affected: the angles of the mouth (in which case the condition may be mistaken for a simple angular cheilitis) and, as in this patient, the external ear.

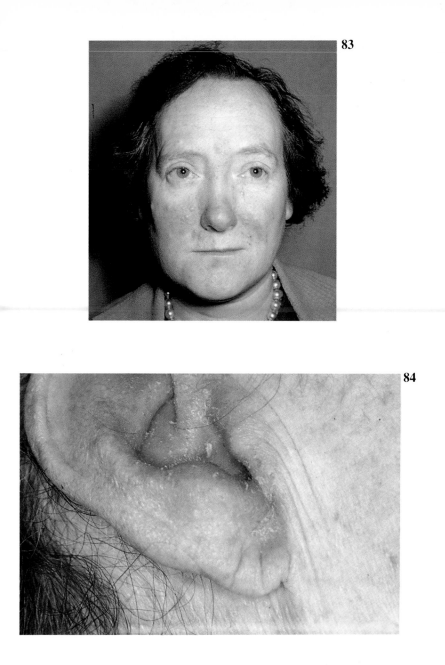

83

84

85 Discoid lupus erythematosus A connective tissue disease that regularly produces orofacial lesions is chronic discoid lupus erythematosus. The mucosal lesions often closely resemble lichen planus, but the facial skin lesions — although not always easy to recognize — present as more diffuse scaly red patches that often also affect the lips. The facial lesions often first appear following exposure to bright sunlight. The histological appearance is not always clearly differentiated from that of lichen planus, and diagnosis following biopsy may not be easy. The lesion in **85**, across the bridge of the nose, is characteristic.

86 Self inflicted trauma If inexplicable excoriated lesions appear on the face, the possibility of dermatitis artefacta — self inflicted trauma — should be considered. This may, in extreme cases, be combined with a cheek chewing habit so severe as to cause perforation of the cheek.

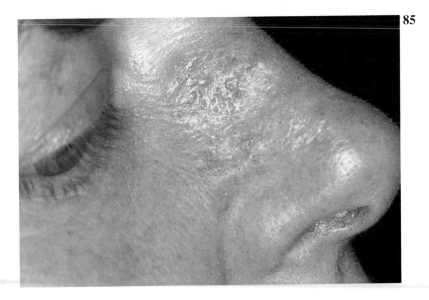

85

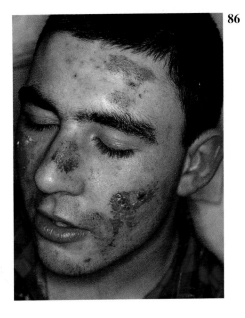

86

87

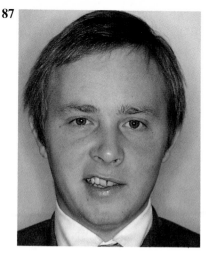

88

87,88 Bell's palsy Both these patients have Bell's palsy, an acute unilateral paralysis of the facial muscles of unknown origin. This is a lower motor neurone lesion, the essential abnormality (whatever it might be) occurring peripheral to the pontine facial nucleus. Similar muscle weakness may occur as a result of a wide variety of lesions below the base of the skull including, for instance, lesions in the parotid gland and traumatic lesions. The Ramsay Hunt syndrome (**54**) includes such a lesion brought about by herpes zoster infection. The essential feature of lower motor neurone lesions is that all the facial muscles (including those of the forehead) are affected. In Bell's palsy there may or may not be distortion of taste sensation on the affected side — presumably depending on the precise site of the causative lesion in relation to the chorda tympani nerve.

Infections of the oral mucosa

The oral mucosa shows a remarkably low susceptibility to infection: particularly, bacterial infection. This is probably due to the protective nature of the saliva, which contains a number of antibacterial substances. It is when the immune system is defective that bacterial lesions of the oral mucosa and lips become significant. Examples have been given in **56** and **57**.

Viral infections of the oral mucosa are, in contrast, relatively common. Primary herpetic stomatitis is the usual first clinical manifestation of the presence of the virus, and does not necessarily imply any immune deficiency, except against the virus concerned.

Fungal infections, in particular by candidal species, are also not uncommon. The organisms are present in the oral cavities of a high proportion of individuals; when the immune defences are lowered in some way, the organisms become active and clinical infection occurs. At the present time the most often quoted situation in which this occurs is in HIV associated conditions. There are, however, many other abnormalities of the immune system and of other bodily functions (such as the haematological and endocrine systems) that may result in the lowering of defences against infection. Oral candidiasis is almost always the result of some such situation.

For reasons of clinical convenience, the oral lesions in HIV disease (**108–111**) are grouped together in this section.

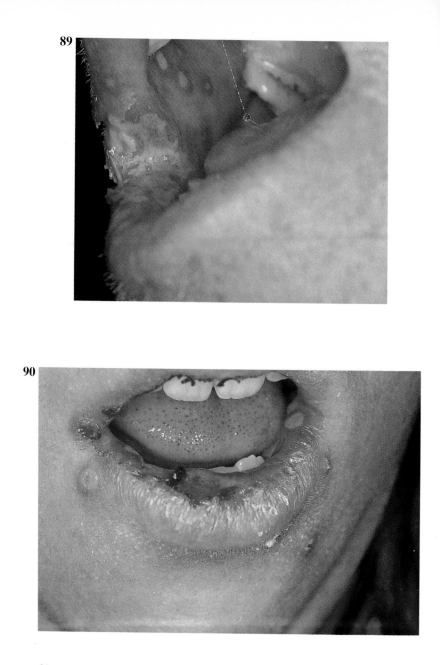

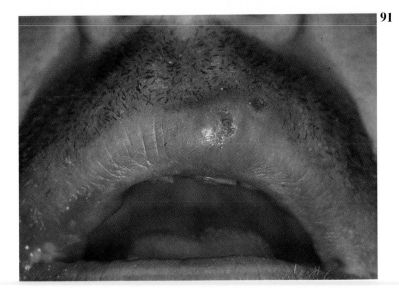

89,90,91,92   Acute herpetic stomatitis   Acute herpetic stomatitis represents a primary infection by the herpes simplex virus. Whatever the immune response may be, a further acute herpetic stomatitis is almost unknown. The primary infection may occur at almost any age and may affect the whole of the oral mucosa and circumoral tissues, with the production of vesicles that rapidly break down to produce shallow ulcers. In child patients in particular, the gingivae may be inflamed and swollen (**92**). Primary herpetic lesions, mostly affecting the perioral tissues, have also been shown in **47–49**.

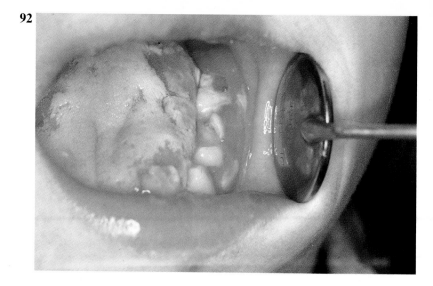

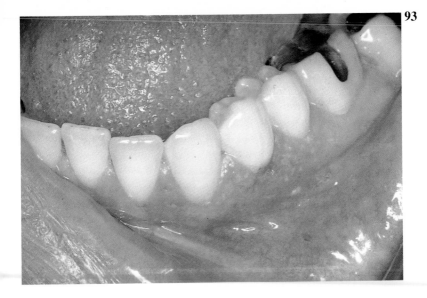

93 Recurrent intraoral herpetic lesions Recurrent labial and perioral herpes (**50–51**) is very common. However, recurrent intraoral herpetic lesions are extremely rare. Shown here is a group of ruptured gingival recurrent herpetic lesions — the diagnosis has been confirmed by studies of the vesicle fluid. It is not known why a very few patients should be susceptible to such lesions. The occurrence of these lesions on the gingivae is common to all reported cases.

94   Thrush   Acute pseudomembranous candidiasis (thrush) is (in all but very young babies with an undeveloped immune system) a sign of a debilitating generalized disease. *Candida* species are effectively commensal in the normal mouth; but, in a wide variety of generalized diseases that result in the lowering of immunological surveillance, the *Candida* may proliferate to produce the superficial pseudomembrane of thrush. Haematological conditions, diabetes mellitus and many other generalized abnormalities may first show up in this way. Many other white patches of the oral mucosa are wrongly initially diagnosed as being of thrush.

95   Thrush   This further example of acute pseudomembranous candidiasis, occurring on the tongue of a patient with an adrenal tumour, bears a remarkable resemblance to many of the illustrations of hairy leukoplakia, the AIDS related lesion described below.

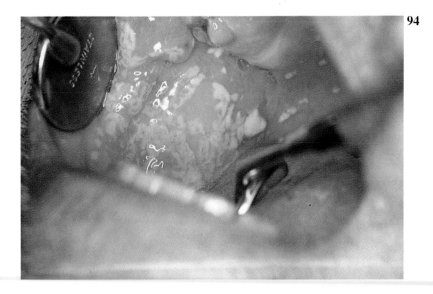

94

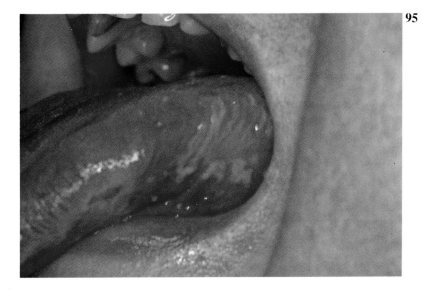

95

96   Chronic mucocutaneous candidiasis   Shown is the tongue of a patient with chronic mucocutaneous candidiasis. This is a condition, which may or may not be genetically determined, in which there is a widespread candidiasis affecting mucous membranes as well as the skin and its appendages (particularly the finger nails). In some patients there are associated endocrine disorders: the endocrine candidiasis syndrome. Although there is clearly a lack of immune protection against candidal invasion, primary immune deficiencies are not always easy to demonstrate. A number of classifications have been proposed according to the clinical and genetic factors involved. The introduction of safer systemically acting antifungal drugs seems likely to revolutionize the outlook for these patients.

97   Acute atrophic candidiasis   This is acute atrophic candidiasis affecting the tongue and associated with candidal angular cheilitis. This has followed a course of antibiotic treatment that has led to overgrowth of the normal oral candidal flora (antibiotic sore tongue). This is the most painful form of oral candidiasis; in other forms discomfort is minimal. It often follows on long-term steroid therapy, as well as the use of antibiotics. It is particularly likely to occur in those patients given local antibiotic–steroid therapy for oral lesions of such conditions as pemphigus and major erosive lichen planus. Prophylactic antifungal therapy eliminates this side effect.

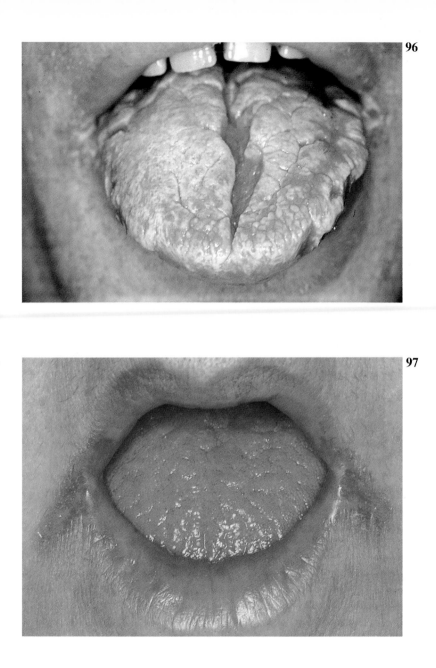

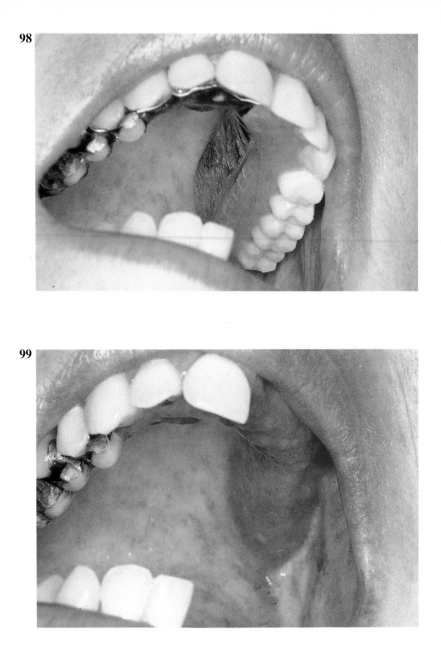

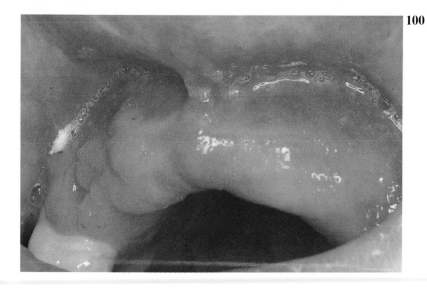

98,99,100 Chronic atrophic candidiasis Chronic atrophic candidiasis is a painless condition that occurs in the palatal tissues under dentures, either partial (**98,99**) or full (**100**), that have been worn continuously. This is by far the most common form of oral candidiasis, occurring in 24% of all denture wearers. Its fiery red appearance accounts for its otherwise entirely unsuitable name of denture sore mouth.

101,102 Chronic hyperplastic candidiasis Shown is chronic hyperplastic candidiasis, also known as candida leukoplakia. The precise relationship between the Candidal invasion of the epithelium and the hyperplastic epithelial changes seen in these lesions is the subject of much speculation. However, there is no doubt that such lesions have a high potential for malignant transformation. As is often the case, the patient with this buccal lesion also had bilateral *Candida*-infected angular cheilitis (**102**).

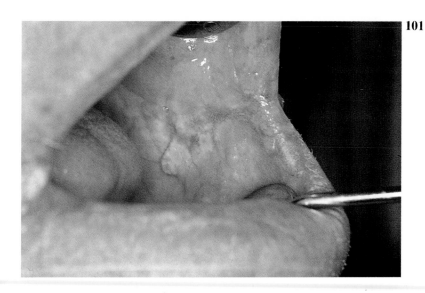

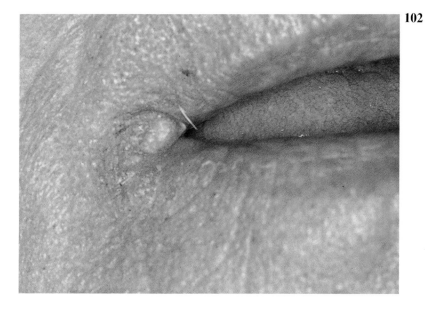

103 Chronic hyperplastic candidiasis Shown is a patient after gastrectomy with unsatisfactory follow up monitoring. On haematological screening he was found to be iron, folate and B_{12} deficient. The lesions on the dorsum of the tongue were of chronic hyperplastic candidiasis with an added superficial candidal pseudomembrane.

104 Primary syphilis Apart from the relatively common acute ulcerative gingivitis (shown below in the section on the teeth and gingivae), intraoral bacterial infections of the mucosa are relatively rare. A classic example is primary syphilis. The lesion in **104** is a chancre (primary syphilitic lesion) of the tongue.

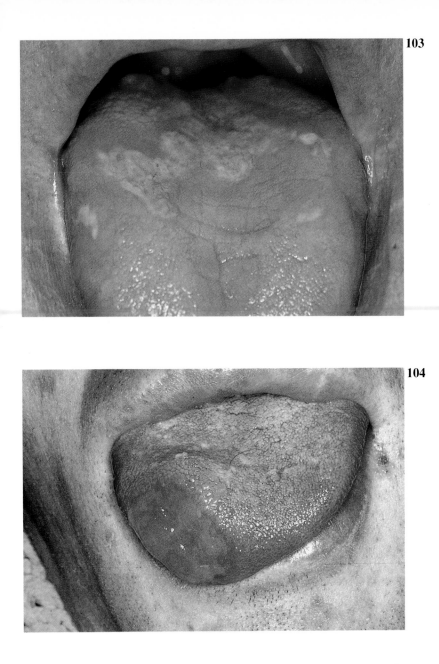

105

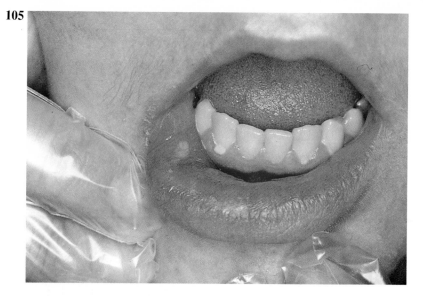

106

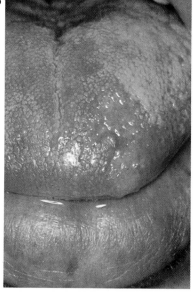

105,106 Secondary syphilis This apparently innocuous ulcer of the lower lip (**105**) is a secondary syphilitic lesion. An even less suspicious lesion of the tongue that is also a secondary syphilitic lesion is shown in **106**.

107 Tertiary syphilis Shown is the classical tertiary syphilitic tongue, virtually never seen now as a result of the generally successful treatment of early syphilis. The patient's tongue shows leukoplakia and areas of malignant change. There is no clear explanation for this situation; it has been suggested that it is a result of the depression of the cell mediated immune response and, hence, of the immune surveillance mechanism in the patients involved.

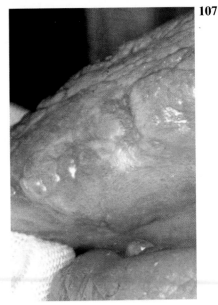

83

108 AIDS: Oral thrush Oral thrush (acute pseudomembranous candidiasis) in a patient with AIDS is shown. Oral candidiasis is a common feature of HIV disease, particularly in the later stages when AIDS has developed or is about to develop. Acute pseudomembranous candidiasis is an important indicator of the possibility of HIV disease in patients in whom no other systemic predisposing factor for the infection can be recognized.

109 AIDS: Hairy leukoplakia Hairy lekoplakia is the term used to describe this corrugated form of leukoplakia, which affects the lateral margins of the tongue in HIV positive patients. The original term used to describe this lesion was hairy cell leukoplakia, descriptive of the histological features of the lesion rather than its clinical appearance. This is not a candida leukoplakia, but it has been suggested that the Epstein–Barr virus is implicated in its aetiology. Recently, however, the electron microscopic evidence for this has been questioned. At the time of writing the precise aetiology of this lesion must be considered questionable. This lesion is not considered as having significant premalignant potential.

110 AIDS: Periodontal disease Rapidly destructive periodontal disease is seen in some patients with HIV disease. The reason for this is not clear, but it presumably represents an exaggeration of the effects of infective agents involved in the periodontitis as a result of immunosuppression.

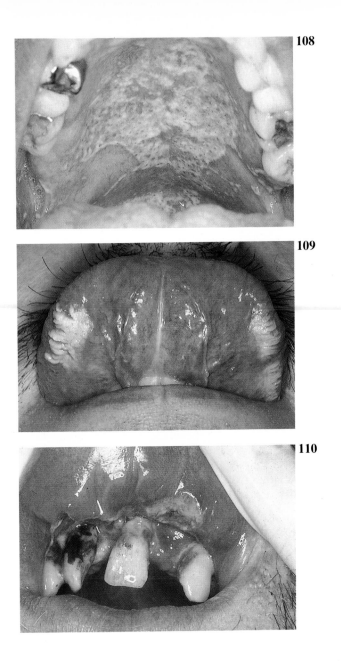

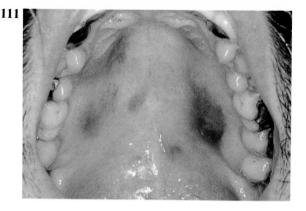

111 AIDS: Kaposi's sarcoma Kaposi's sarcoma of the palate in AIDS. This lesion was described long ago as a rare dermatological lesion, relatively benign and usually affecting the lower limbs. It is, however, found in a much more aggressive form in AIDS patients, often appearing on the palatal mucosa as part of a diffuse and multicentric condition that may extend to many bodily structures. It is currently thought to derive from vascular endothelial cells. These dusky macular lesions conform to the usual description, although more proliferative lesions also occur.

Aphthous ulcers

The term aphthous ulceration is used to describe a group of conditions of unknown aetiology that commonly affect the oral mucosa. Although there is a wide spectrum of clinical behaviour, there are three accepted variants:

- Minor aphthous ulcers are relatively small, occur most commonly in a cyclic pattern and heal (without scar formation) in some ten to 14 days.
- Major aphthous ulcers are generally larger than the minor variety, last longer (sometimes for many weeks) and often heal with scarring,
- Herpetiform ulcers are in general the smallest variety of these ulcers but are often multiple and may coalesce to form larger ulcers. They are the most common form of these ulcers to be associated with nutritional deficiencies.

Any of these forms of oral ulceration (but particularly major aphthous ulceration) may be associated with the multisystem disorders of Behçet's syndrome. Anterior uveitis (121) is the most common ocular disorder in this syndrome. Oral and genital ulceration may be associated with ocular, vasculitic, neurological, arthritic and other abnormalities in this condition. Of these, the oral ulceration is the most consistant feature.

112 Aphthous ulcer of the lower lip   A solitary aphthous ulcer of the lower lip. The size is characteristic, although they can be considerably larger. The definition of minor as distinct from major aphthous ulceration depends much more on the duration of the ulcers than on their size.

113 Minor aphthous ulcers   This is a group of minor aphthous ulcers on a characteristic site: the lateral margins of the tongue. The group shows some size variation, but all are within the usual limits expected in minor aphthous ulceration. The coated tongue is a secondary effect due to stasis resulting from the discomfort of the ulcers.

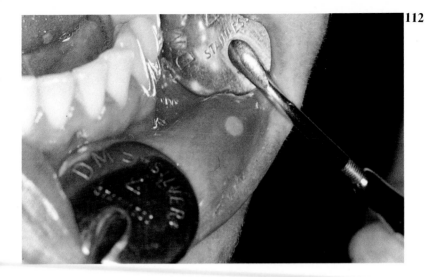

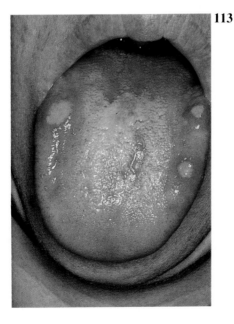

89

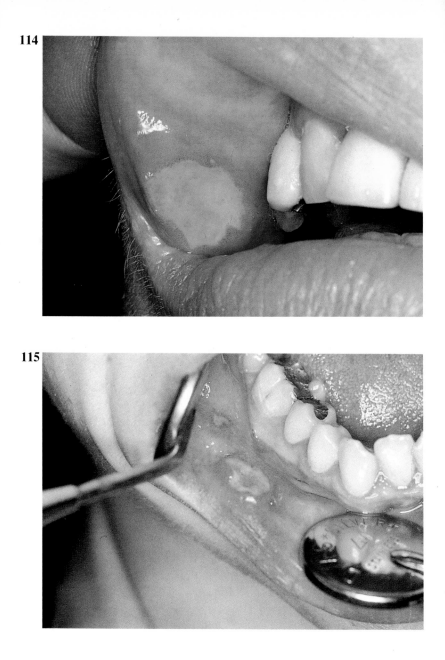

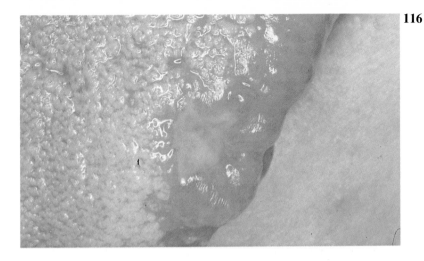

114,115,116,117,118 Major aphthous ulcers Major aphthous ulcers affecting various sites are shown. One of the consequences of the long duration of the ulcers is a much more indurated margin to the lesions than in the case of minor ulcers. An ulcer such as that in **116** may easily be mistaken for a malignant lesion if the history of recurrent ulceration is not recognized.

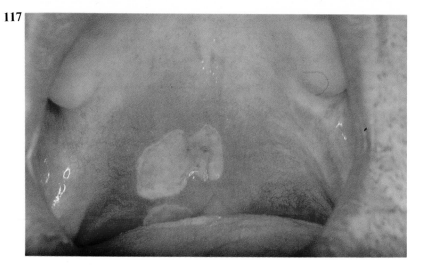

117

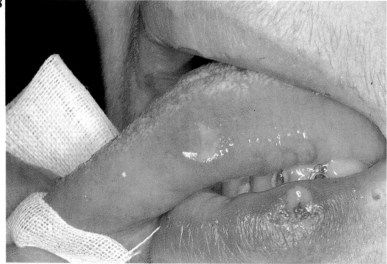

118

119 Major aphthous ulcers
Major aphthous ulceration often affects the lips and, particularly, the commissures. There may be considerable scar formation and consequent tissue distortion (**119**). A characteristic feature of major aphthous ulceration, however, is its tendency to affect the posterior part of the mouth and the oropharynx.

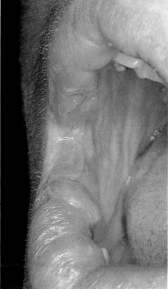

119

120 Herpetiform ulcers Shown is a group of herpetiform ulcers on the lateral margin of the tongue. As is often the case, some have coalesced to form larger ulcers, and the whole group is set against an erythematous background.

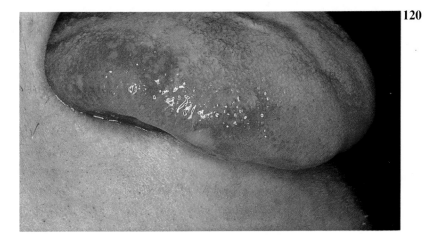

120

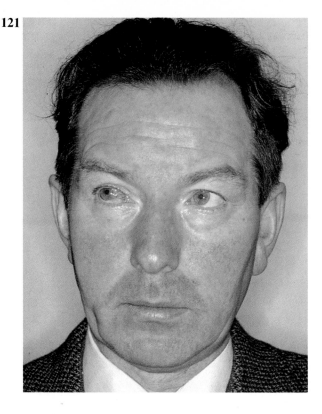

121 Behçet's syndrome A patient who suffers from Behçet's syndrome with ulcers of the oral and genital mucosa, joint lesions and vasculitic problems. The erythematous skin rash and reddening of the right eye due to an anterior uveitis are evident.

White patches of the oral mucosa

The term white patch implies a lesion of the oral mucosa in which there has been an abnormality of the maturation process and, hence, of keratinization. The term leukoplakia, although apparently similar, has a slightly different implication. The WHO definition of leukoplakia is of a white patch on the oral mucosa that cannot be wiped off and is not susceptible to any other clinical diagnosis. Leukoplakia is a condition that is often considered to be essentially premalignant, but this is by no means necessarily so. Nonetheless, a statistically assessable proportion of lesions clinically diagnosed as leukoplakia will eventually undergo malignant transformation.

It will be seen that there is a transition between the conditions seen in this section under the heading "White patches" and some of those seen in the next section under the heading "Oral lesions in diseases of the skin": in particular, the oral lesions of lichen planus. Differential diagnosis of these conditions is highly dependent on biopsy study.

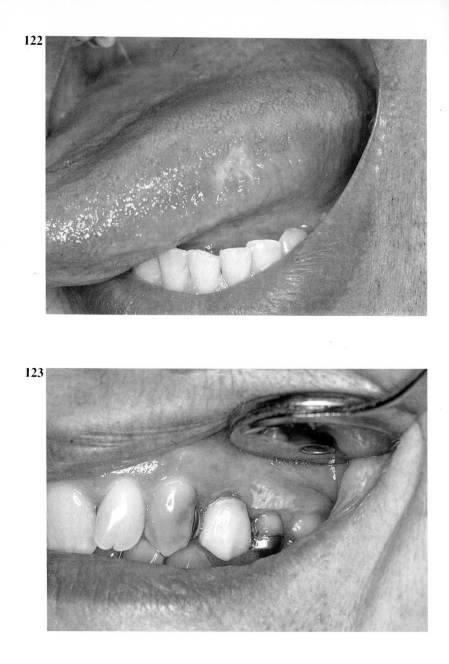

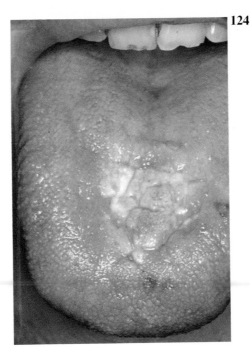

122,123,124 Leukoplakia These are three examples of leukoplakia of the lateral margin of the tongue (**122**), the gingivae (**123**) and the dorsum of the tongue (**124**). These restricted lesions are of no known origin, although frictional trauma might be suggested in each case. All three of these lesions showed entirely innocuous histological features on biopsy. Biopsy is virtually mandatory: clinical assessment alone is, even in highly experienced hands, a doubtful procedure.

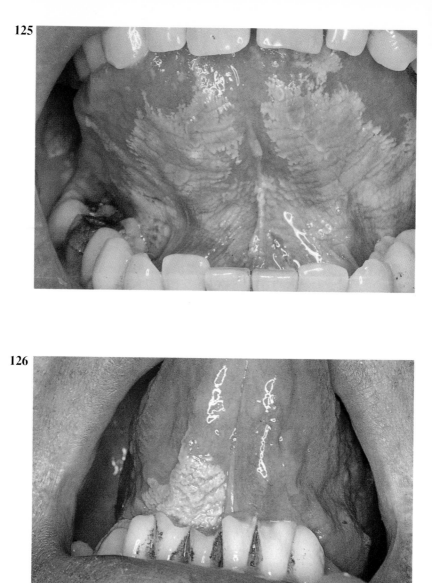

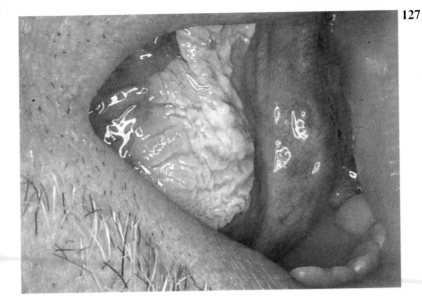

125,126,127 Leukoplakia Leukoplakia of the floor of the mouth and the dorsal surface of the tongue was at one time thought to be of insignificant premalignant potential. White lesions in this site were generally thought to be naevi with no malignant tendencies. However, as the result of a number of recent retrospective histological studies, the concept of the floor of mouth leukoplakia as a lesion with high malignant potential has come to the fore. The lesions show the typical "ebbing tide" appearance often associated with leukoplakia in this site.

128 Floor of mouth leukoplakia This lesion, described in the previous edition of this atlas as an example of a non hereditary epithelial naevus would now, in the light of contemporary knowledge, be regarded with suspicion as a potentially malignant lesion, whatever the histology might initially indicate.

129 Lesion with epithelial dysplasia This lesion, with a more irregular appearance than those shown in **125–127** and with some nearby areas of epithelial atrophy, showed considerable epithelial dysplasia on biopsy.

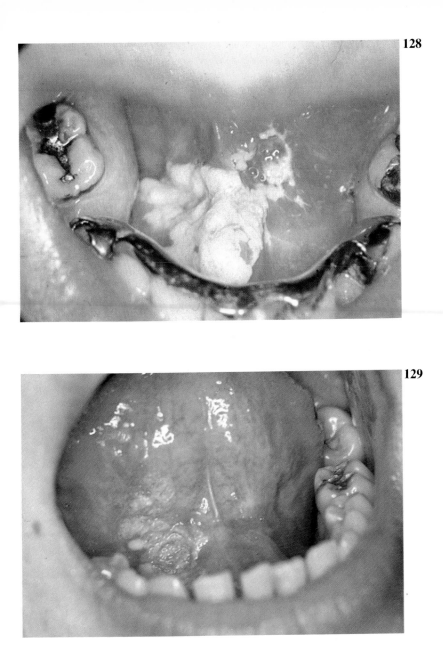

130

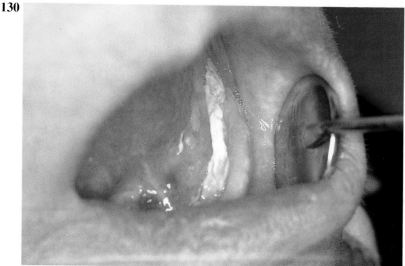

130 Floor of mouth leukoplakia A densely white floor of mouth leukoplakia with aggressive histological features. In spite of surgical treatment and careful monitoring, a carcinoma eventually developed in this site.

131,132 Candida leukoplakia Both these lesions were found, on biopsy, to have an infiltration of candidal hyphae in the epithelium. The relationship of *Candida* to the formation of leukoplakias is not fully understood: it is not known whether there is a causal relationship or whether the fungae are secondary invaders. It is thought, however, that the infected lesions (*Candida leukoplakias*) are more likely to undergo malignant transformation than are non Candidal lesions.

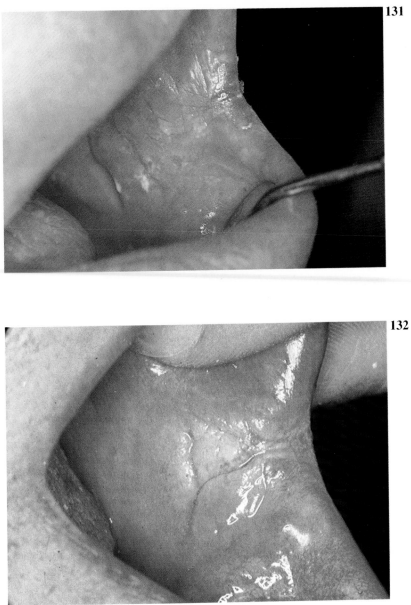

131

132

133

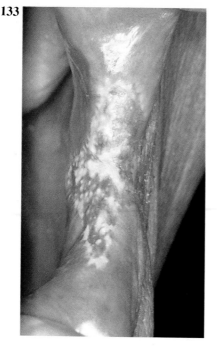

133 Erythroplakia This lesion has areas of red atrophic mucosa (erythroplakia) associated with leukoplakia. Erythroplakia is often found on biopsy to have a high incidence of epithelial atypia, and such lesions have a high potential for malignant transformation.

134,135 Speckled leukoplakia Both the lesions shown are of speckled leukoplakia — intermediate between erythroplakia and leukoplakia. It has been suggested that the term speckled erythroplakia would be more suitable since the incidence of malignant transformation in such lesions is comparable to that of erythroplakia and, thus, higher than that in homogenous leukoplakias. The site at the commissure is characteristic, and *Candida* are often seen on biopsy.

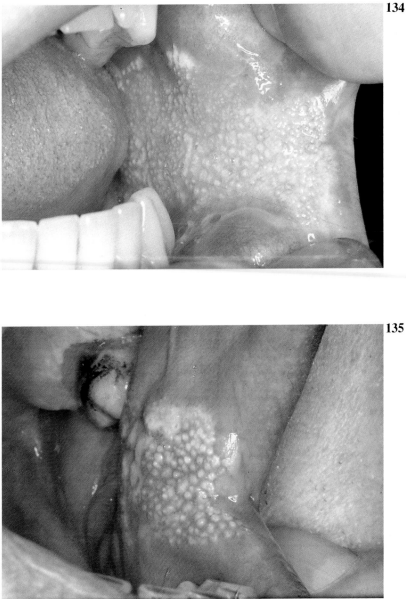

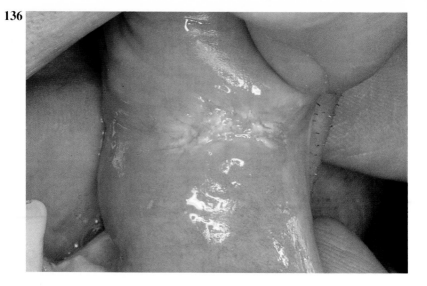

136 Commissural leukoplakia Shown is a leukoplakia of the buccal mucosa close to the commissure in a heavy smoker. Biopsy showed the presence of *Candida* and of marked epithelial atypia. This is characteristic of the so called "smoker's keratosis". Many candidal leukoplakias in heavy smokers arise in this site.

137 "Pipe smoker's palate" Changes in the palatal mucosa associated with smoking — and particularly with pipe smoking — result in a faint all-over whitening of the palatal mucosa. The mucous glands enlarge and become prominent while their ducts dilate to produce a central red spot. This is a typical example of the so called pipe smoker's palate (nicotinic stomatitis). It is suggested that the lesion is the result of the direction of the tobacco smoke from the pipe onto the palate. Oddly enough, the overall behaviour of lesions such as this indicates a low premalignant potential.

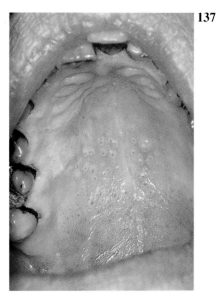

137

138 "Pipe smoker's palate" In a few cases of pipe smoker's palate there may be more widespread inflammatory changes in one or more of the palatal glands with consequent tissue breakdown and chronic ulceration. This is a very unusual gross example.

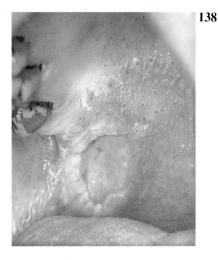

138

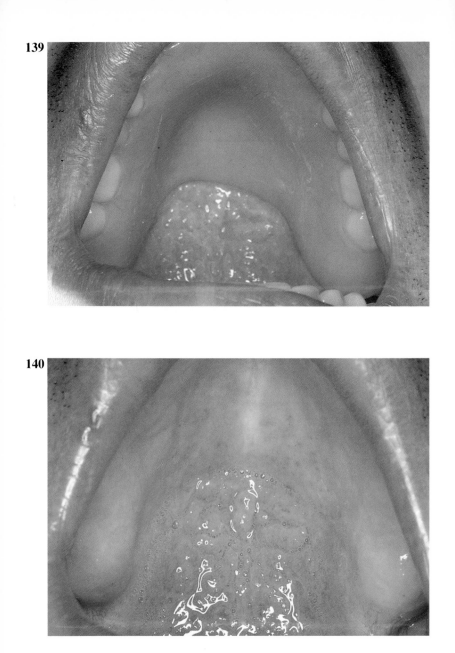

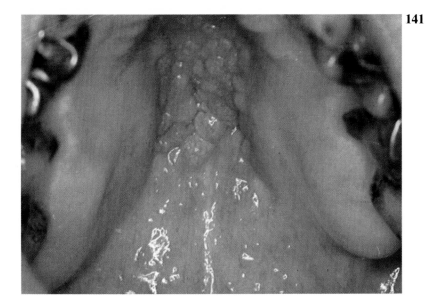

139,140,141 Papillary hyperplasia of the palate Papillary
hyperplasia of the palate is a superficially similar lesion to that of a
smoker's keratosis, but there is not the same relationship between the
mucous glands and the numerous papilloma-like lesions on the palatal
mucosa. In the patient shown in **139** and **140**, the lesion occurs behind
the line of the denture. This patient was a pipe smoker. In other
patients papillary hyperplasia may occur under a denture, as in **141**,
where the whole palate was covered by a denture replacing one tooth.
It would seem likely that various forms of irritation may result in
lesions of this kind.

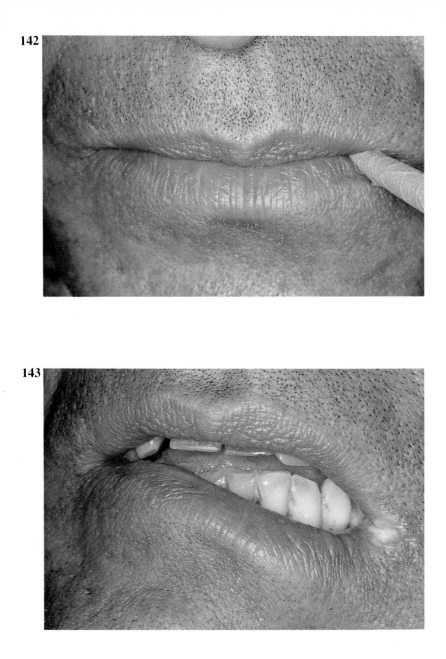

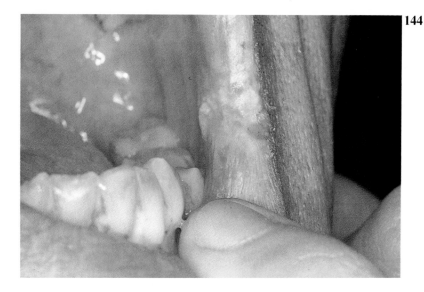

142,143,144 Tobacco induced leukoplakia A localized area of keratosis may occur in response to tobacco smoke in various circumstances. The lesion of the commissure shown here is characteristic of those resulting from bidi smoking. A bidi is a form of Indian cigarette that is associated with a high incidence of leukoplakia.

145 Frictional keratosis Lesions such as the frictional keratosis shown are often seen on the buccal mucosa. There is often some form of habit involved, although this may be quite unrecognized by the patient. These lesions are not regarded as having a significant malignant potential.

146 Traumatic ulcer of the tongue Shown is a typical traumatic ulcer of the tongue, caused by friction from the orthodontic wiring on the lower teeth. Acute traumatic ulcers frequently have a whitened epithelial margin such as this. It is not a sign of malignancy.

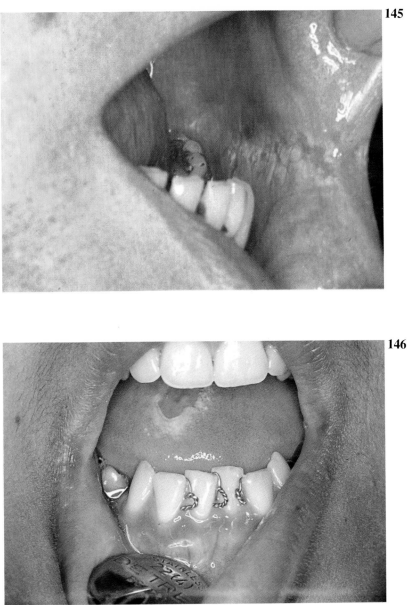

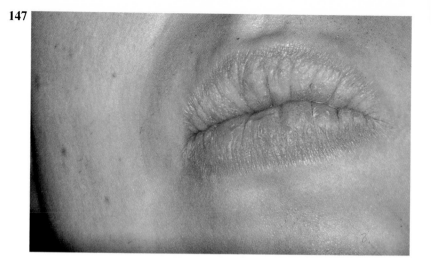

147,148 Cheek chewing lesions Cheek chewing habits (**147**) often result in lesions such as that shown in **148**. The surface of the mucosa becomes rough and partially detached, with small denuded areas where the epithelium has been bitten away.

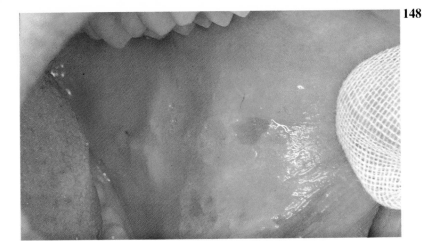

149 Tertiary syphilis This is a further example of the now rare tertiary syphilitic tongue (see also **107**). There are areas of leuko-plakia and of erythroplakia. The malignant potential is high.

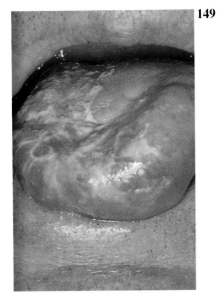

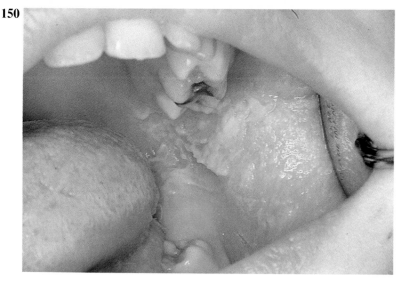

150 Genetically determined white lesions of oral mucosa There are a number of genetically determined white lesions of the oral mucosa. They may affect the oral mucosa alone, a number of mucous membranes, or mucous membranes together with the skin and its appendages. In many of these complex dermal–mucosal syndromes there are similar oral mucosal lesions. This patient has the best known of these conditions: leukokeratosis (or white sponge naevus). The rather bluish appearance of the affected mucosa is due to the presence of many large clear cells in the epithelium: again, a common factor in a number of these rare conditions. Even in this relatively well studied condition the genetic basis is uncertain and, probably, variable. It is considered to have no malignant potential.

151 Aspirin burn in the buccal sulcus This is a well known but often misdiagnosed condition: a burn caused by placing an aspirin tablet in the buccal sulcus next to a tooth in order to relieve toothache. This is still a common practice. The combination of acute onset, the previous history of toothache and the proximity of the lesion to a suspect tooth should indicate the true diagnosis.

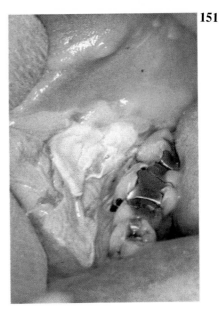

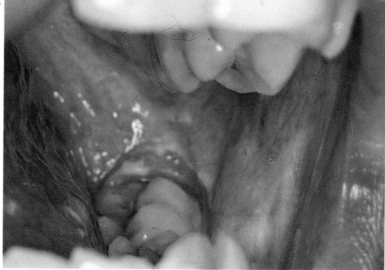

152 Submucous fibrosis Submucous fibrosis is a condition largely, but not entirely, confined to the Indian subcontinent. Excessive amounts of collagen are laid down in the corium of the oral mucosa, leading to loss of flexibility in the tissues, difficulty in opening the mouth, and binding down of the tongue. The oral epithelium undergoes atrophic change, initially leading to minor ulceration but later with the formation of leukoplakias showing a high incidence of epithelial atypia. The rather marbled appearance of the oral mucosa is shown, together with surface irregularities due to the formation of collagen bundles. Recent work indicates a genetic basis to the condition (via the HLA mechanism), although hypersensitivity reactions may also be involved. This is considered to be a lesion with a high potential for malignant change.

Oral lesions in diseases of the skin

The behaviour of the oral mucous membrane in its response to disease processes lies between that of the skin and that of the gastrointestinal mucosa. In view of its embryonic origin, this is not surprising.

Oral lesions in skin diseases may clinically resemble those of the skin (as, for instance in pemphigoid), or may be quite dissimilar (as in lichen planus). Histologically, however, they are very similar, and a biopsy study of oral lesions (particularly using immunofluorescent techniques) may prove very helpful in those situations (such as pemphigus) in which the oral lesions may appear first.

For reasons of clinical compatibility some lesions not associated with skin diseases are included in this section.

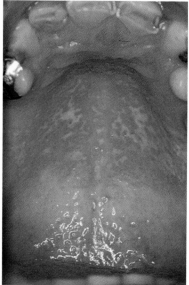

153,154,155,156 Lichen planus
Lichen planus is a skin disease in which oral lesions are relatively common. The oral lesions may occur at the same time as the skin lesions, may precede them, or may follow them. In many patients, therefore, at any given time there may be only oral lesions present. These oral lesions have a wide range of presentation and may be classified in many ways; the present writer uses the broad clinical terms non erosive, minor erosive, and major erosive to describe major variants. These variations in appearance (and also in

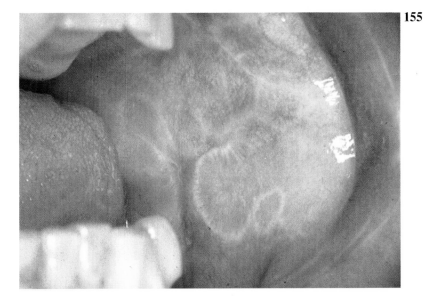

clinical behaviour) may lead to confusion in diagnosis. The histological appearance, however, in all variants resembles that of skin lesions. Biopsy is highly advisable to settle the diagnosis in most cases. The classic appearance of white reticulations of non erosive lichen planus on the buccal mucosa is seen in **153** and a similar appearance on the palatal mucosa in **155**. However, there are many variations in form: a circinate pattern is shown in **156**, and a more plaque like lesion of the tongue in **157**.

156

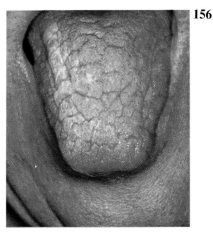

157,158   Minor erosive lichen planus   In minor erosive lichen planus, erosions are formed by the loss of atrophic areas of epithelium such as those seen between the white reticulations in **157**. The erosions may become quite widespread — as in **158** — but there are almost always some remaining associated areas of white mucosa.

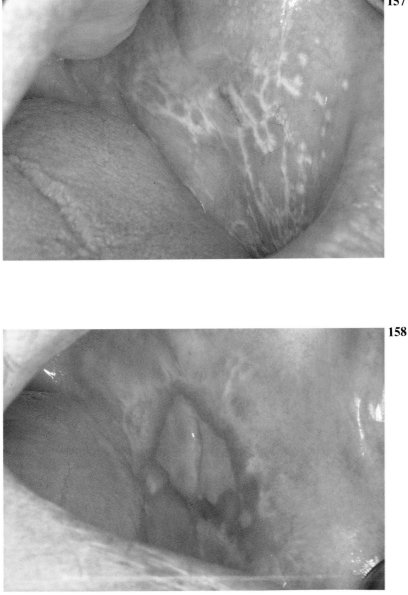

159 Major erosive lichen planus In major erosive lichen planus (**159**) the ulceration tends to be of sudden onset, often not preceded by recognizable non erosive lesions. It most commonly affects the buccal mucosa and, especially, the tongue. The shiny, clearly demarcated ulcer shown here is quite characteristic. Associated white lesions may be less obvious than in the case of minor erosive lichen planus but, nonetheless, are almost always present to some degree.

All forms of lichen planus may occur as a response to drug therapy — the so called lichenoid reaction. The recognition of this is based on the history: there is effectively no difference between drug induced and non drug induced lesions. A wide range of drugs can have this effect; particularly the anti rheumatic drugs and, in particular, the non steroidal anti inflammatory agents. The lesions do not necessarily regress on withdrawal of the drug.

160 Gingival lichen planus Gingival lichen planus may occur in association with other, more widespread, lesions of the mucosa. It may also, however, present effectively without any other lesions, and the clinical diagnosis may be difficult. The erythematous, rather fragile, gingival tissues may (as in this case) show no hint of an origin in an essentially keratotic lesion, although in some cases (usually non erosive) the gingival lesions closely resemble those on other parts of the mucosa. To add to the diagnostic difficulties, pemphigoid may appear in a very similar way. However, this condition, often described as desquamative gingivitis, is most often eventually diagnosed as being a variant of minor erosive lichen planus. Previously it was frequently attributed to hormonal imbalance in female patients.

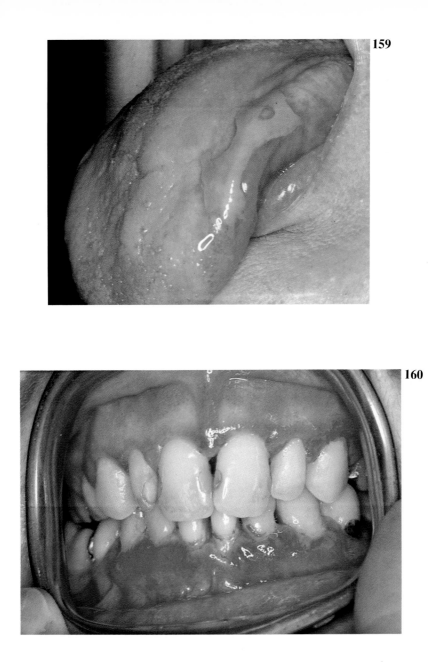

161,162 Pemphigoid Pemphigoid is a variable disease of the skin, the mucous membranes, or both. Nomenclature differs, but it is possible to distinguish two basic conditions: generalized pemphigoid, in which the skin is predominantly affected and the mucous membranes rarely; and mucosal pemphigoid, in which the mucosa are affected with only occasional skin involvement. The essential lesions are subepithelial blisters associated with the deposition of mainly IgG class antibodies along the basal zone. Although the skin lesions may be relatively robust, the oral blisters rapidly break down to leave eroded areas. **161** shows such erosions on the palate, **162** shows them on the gingivae. In neither case is the essentially bullous nature of the disease evident. The patients are predominantly female (4:1).

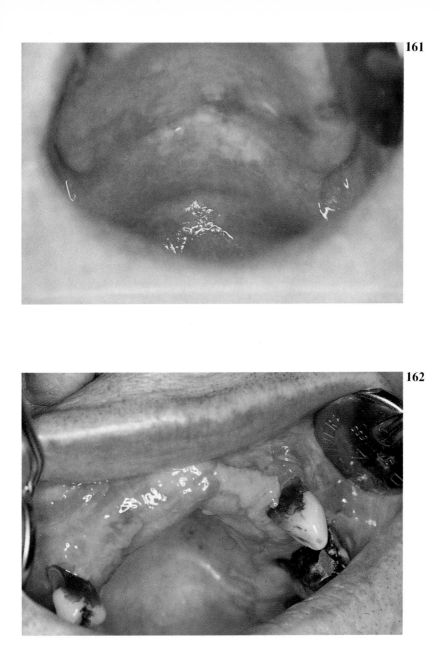

161

162

163 Benign mucous membrane pemphigoid This represents a particular type of pemphigoid, often described as benign mucous membrane pemphigoid, in which the oral lesions particularly affect the soft palate and heal with some degree of scarring. In this, as in other forms of pemphigoid, the conjunctivae are often involved. All patients with pemphigoid of any variety should have a professional eye examination to detect the possible onset of eye lesions.

164 Gingival pemphigoid Gingival pemphigoid may closely resemble gingival lichen planus (**160**). Biopsy of the nearby mucosa, with immunofluorescent studies, may be necessary to determine the differential diagnosis.

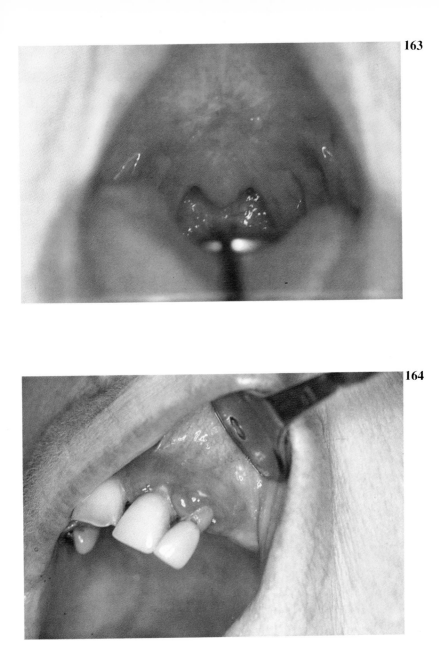

165 Pemphigus The oral lesions in pemphigus have a particular significance, since in 50% of patients they are the first indication of this potentially fatal disease. This is likely to be a lifelong condition for which prolonged steroid treatment may be necessary. The bullous lesions of the oral mucosa are fragile and rapidly break down; the whole of the mouth may be affected by erosions, which may persist even if control of the skin lesions is attained. Widespread scar formation and restriction in opening of the mouth may also occur. Oral hygiene is almost impossible to maintain because of mucosal fragility and the dental treatment of these patients may be very difficult. If an acute bullous disease is suspected, biopsy of an oral lesion with immunofluorescent studies is strongly indicated. IgG class antibodies are found binding on the intercellular structures and cell walls of the stratum spinosum.

166 Chronic discoid lupus erythematosus This is a mucosal lesion in chronic discoid lupus erythematosus (CDLE). In a number of connective tissue diseases, such as CDLE, lesions of the buccal mucosa occur that, both clinically and histologically, may be mistaken for lichen planus. However, immunofluorescent studies of biopsy material make the differential diagnosis much less difficult.

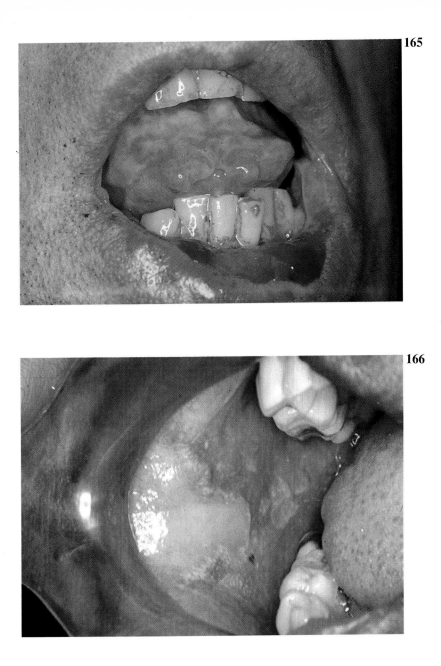

167,168 Erythema multiforme Erythema multiforme is an acute condition affecting skin and mucous membranes with an immunological basis which has not, as yet, been fully defined. It may be a recurrent problem, but may also occur as an isolated episode. Precipitating factors include recurrent herpetic infections and a wide variety of drugs. In many cases, however, there is no evident precipitating factor. As in so many oral conditions, the role of food allergy is now being investigated. The involvement of the lower lip is characteristic (**167**) although the rest of the oral mucosa may also be involved (**168**). The mucosal lesions (which may involve the eyes and genitalia) are essentially fragile bullae that rapidly break down to form erosive areas. The fragility of the bullae is a result of their structure: there is often marked intra-epithelial oedema as well as sub epithelial bulla formation. The intact bulla on the tip of the tongue shown in **168** is very unusual.

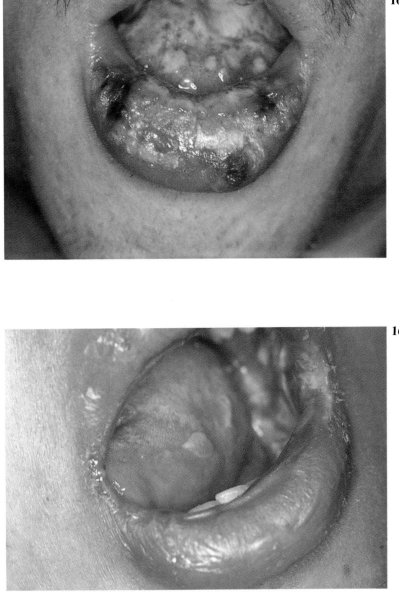

169,170 Blood filled blisters of the oral mucosa Blood filled blisters of the oral mucosa may occur as a result of trauma (as in **169**), in clotting disorders or, in some cases, spontaneously. The occurrence of spontaneous blood blisters in otherwise quite normal patients is well documented; it has been given the unwieldy title, angina bullosa haemorrhagica. The most common site for such blisters is on the soft palate, usually forming when the patient is eating. When the bulla is ruptured there is nothing to distinguish it clinically from other mucosal bullae (**170**). The aetiology of this condition is not known.

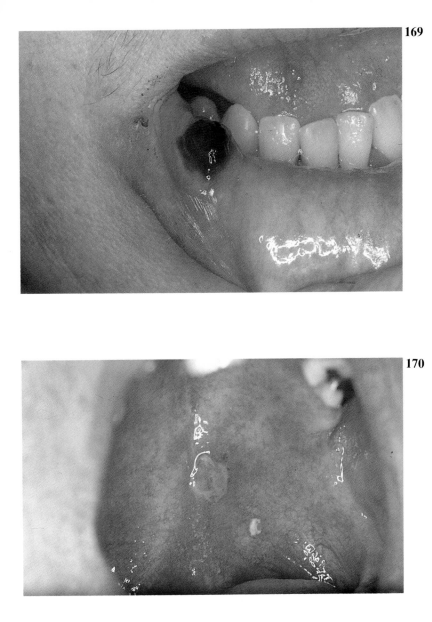

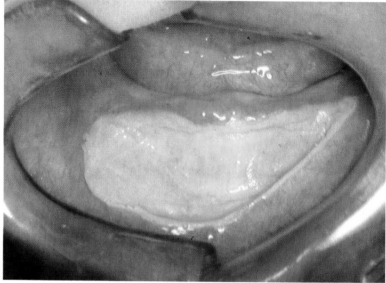

171 Skin graft in the oral mucosa Shown is a skin graft in the oral mucosa (a so called "epithelial inlay") performed as part of a preprosthetic surgical procedure. Even after many years such a graft retains its original appearance and, if biopsied, is found to maintain the histological characteristics of skin, rather than of oral mucosa.

172,173 Stomatitis associated with uraemia A wide range of lesions have been described in patients with advanced renal failure. Of these the most specific is a stomatitis thought to result from biochemical changes in the saliva. This has not been fully investigated, but these illustrations show the condition as it is often described.

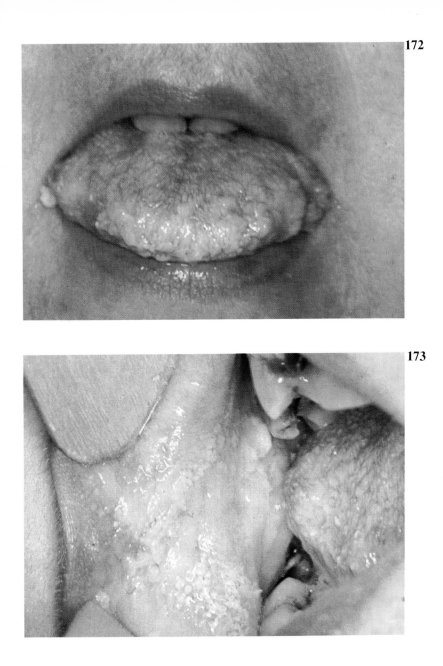

172

173

174,175 Crohn's disease The oral mucosa in Crohn's disease undergoes changes similar to those that occur in the lower gut. There may be folding and "cobblestoning" of the mucosa, with or without primary or secondary ulceration. Biopsy of the affected tissue shows the presence of non caseating tuberculoid granulomas similar to those found in the lower gut. In some few cases it may be necessary to search carefully through many sections to find these granulomas, although in most biopsy specimens there are very large numbers immediately visible. The presence of these granulomatous structures in the mucosa, together with lip or facial swelling (**175**), angular cheilitis and palpable cervical lymph nodes is strongly indicative of Crohn's disease (or of orofacial granulomatosis — a spectrum term favoured by some authorities to include oral Crohn's disease). The erythematous facial skin overlying the swollen areas and shown in **175** is also characteristic, but not always present.

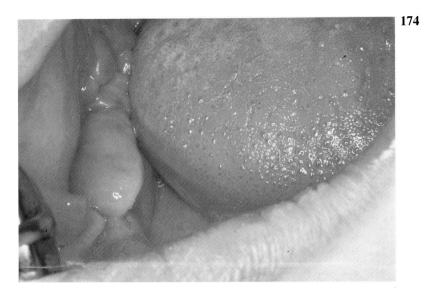

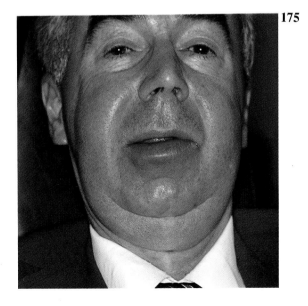

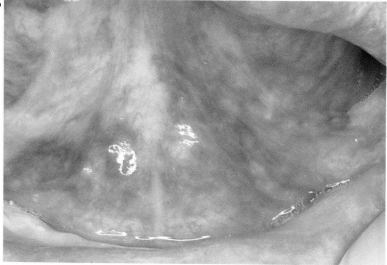

176 Oral mucosal pigmentation Diffuse melanotic pigmentation of the oral mucosa may have many origins. The most famous generalized disease association is that with Addison's disease; the patient shown is an example. Many other endocrine disturbances might result in similar oral pigmentation. However, by far the most common cause of oral mucosal pigmentation is ethnic, and there are several examples of this in various parts of this atlas. A much less well documented source of oral pigmentation is the response to keratotic lesions of various kinds. Lichen planus, in particular, may result in the deposition of clinically recognizable melanin deposits beneath the white epithelial lesions.

Neoplasms and overgrowths of the oral mucosa

The oral cavity is the site for a large number of neoplastic and inflammatory overgrowths. Of these, the most significant in terms of incidence and prognosis is squamous cell carcinoma. This neoplasm shows wide geographical variations in incidence dependent on a wide range of factors, the most often investigated being the use of tobacco in various forms. Many of the inflammatory lesions seen on the oral mucosa are essentially responses to trauma of some kind; the fibro-epithelial polyp (**181**) and the denture granuloma (**182**) are common examples of this.

Although clinical diagnosis, based on appearance, may be the first diagnostic indicator for these lesions, the definitive diagnosis depends on histological study of biopsy material.

177,178 Papillomas of the oral mucosa Papillomas of the oral mucosa may occur on almost any site and in all ages of patients. They are said to have a cauliflower like appearance; and, in fact, some do (**177**). There is virtually no danger of malignant transformation. These two papillomas — of the lingual frenum and the commissure — show quite characteristic features. Papilloma like lesions around the mouth in children are often the result of viral wart transmission following the chewing of warts of the fingers.

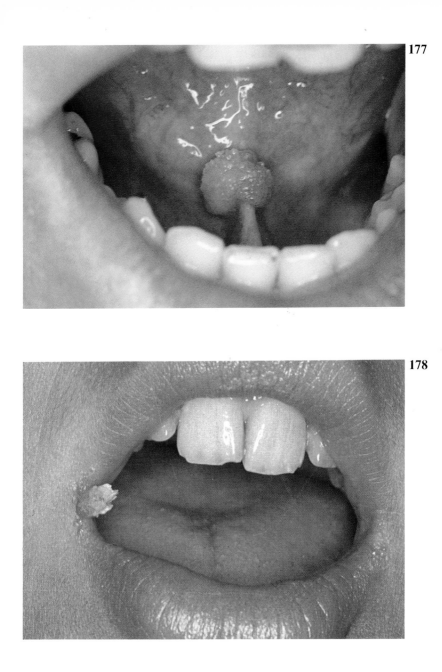

179,180 Papilloma of the palate This flat lesion of the palate, occurring below a denture, has many descriptions, from papilloma to leaf fibroma. It is certainly not a fibroma, but the classification as either a papilloma or a fibro-epithelial polyp can be argued. The proportion of epithelial to connective tissue present argues for an essentially epithelial origin, but this may be a result of the physically constricting environment. When in place on the palatal tissues (**180**) these lesions may be difficult to identify.

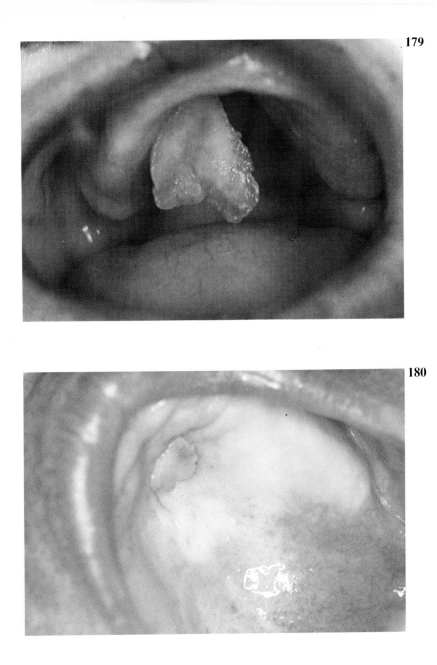

181 Fibro-epithelial polyp The fibro-epithelial polyp shown is in a quite characteristic site: the commissure, where friction from the teeth may occur. The white area on the surface, not always present, is a further mark of this lesion's origin as a result of chronic, mild, frictional trauma. These lesions are entirely benign.

182 Fibroma of the oral cavity A true fibroma of the oral cavity, such as this lesion, is a rare occurrence. The title — implying a benign true neoplasm involving fibroblasts — is often wrongly applied to essentially inflammatory lesions.

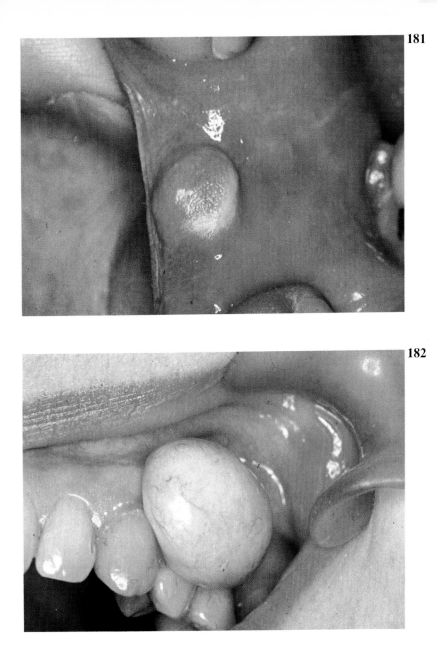

183,184   Denture granuloma   A denture granuloma is essentially the same lesion as a fibro-epithelial polyp, although its appearance is modified by the site of its origin: at the margin of an old, ill fitting denture. Just as in the case of the fibro-epithelial polyp, this is essentially a connective tissue response to chronic trauma. This also is a lesion with virtually no premalignant potential.

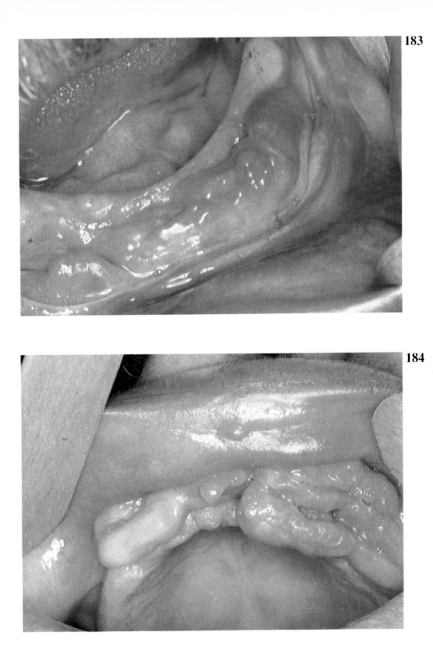

183

184

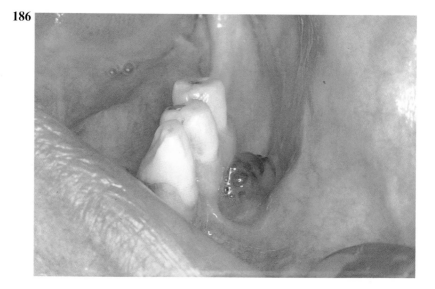

185,186,187,188,189,190 Haemangiomas of the oral soft tissues
Haemangiomas of the oral soft tissues are essentially hamartomas
rather than true neoplasms. This implies that they result from a
dynamic imbalance in the peripheral blood vessels, which leads to

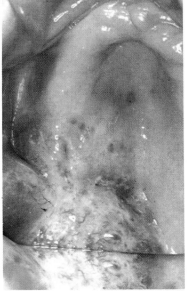

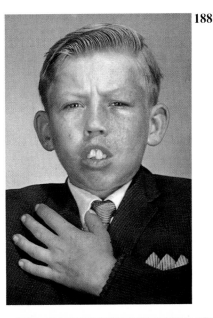

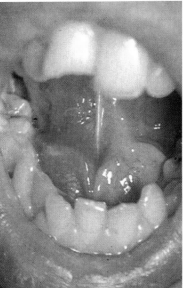

expansion and the production of multiple blood filled spaces in the tissues. Even the rare central haemangiomas that occasionally occur in the facial bones probably have a similar origin; although, because of their site, they are potentially much more dangerous. **185** shows a simple haemangioma of the tongue, a common site. The site of the buccal lesion in **186** is less common. Occasionally, widespread lesions such as that shown in **187** may occur affecting, in this case, the cheek, soft palate and pharyngeal wall. In some patients oropharyngeal haemangiomas may be associated with cerebral and skin lesions of the same kind as in the Sturge–Weber

190

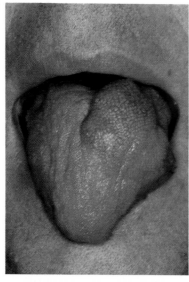

syndrome (**188,189**). Some deep seated haemangiomas of the tongue may have a deceptively non vascular superficial appearance (**190**).

191

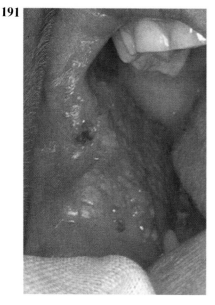

191 Lymphangiomas Lymphangiomas of the orofacial tissues are not a particular rarity. They resemble haemangiomas in their consistency and surface appearance, but evidently contain clear fluid rather than blood. Like haemangiomas, these are essentially hamartomas rather than neoplasms, although they may grow with age. In some instances the lesion may contain both expanded lymphatics and blood vessels (a lymphhaemangioma).

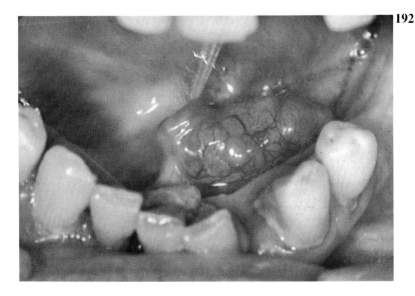

192 Pleomorphic adenoma Salivary gland neoplasms may arise in major and minor salivary glands in virtually any site in the orofacial region. The pleomorphic adenoma shown here is arising in the sublingual gland.

193,194 Pleomorphic adenomas   These are pleomorphic adenomas occurring in their most common site of minor salivary gland origin: the junction of the hard and soft palates, where there are many minor glands. The single lobule shown in **193** is more common than the multilobulated structure in **194**.

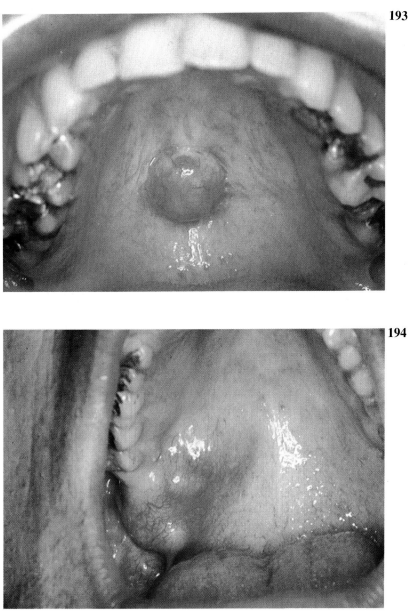

193

194

195   Ulcerated salivary gland neoplasm   Although it is virtually impossible to assess the nature of salivary gland tumours without histological study, ulceration is often a marker of the more aggressive lesions, which may behave in an entirely malignant manner.

196   Giant cell granuloma   A range of granulomatous lesions may occur at any site in the oral mucosa, although lesions of this kind are much more common on the gingivae. The fibro-epithelial polyp is one member of this broad spectrum of inflammatory lesions, which also includes the so called pyogenic granuloma. In the case of the fibro-epithelial polyp, however, there is usually much clearer evidence of the action of mechanical trauma as an initiating factor for the lesion. The example shown is a relative rarity: a peripheral giant cell granuloma in an edentulous patient.

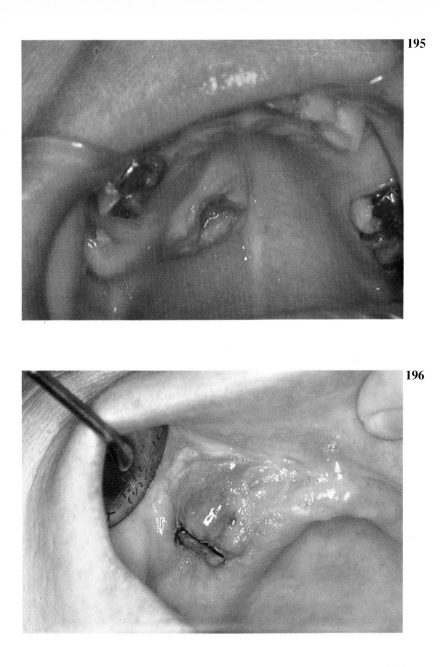

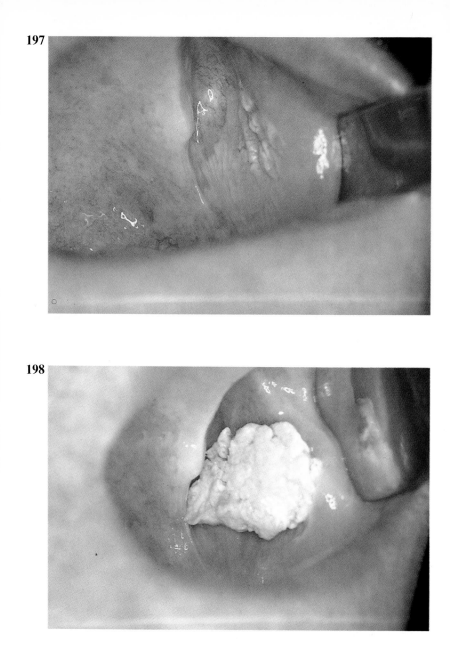

197, 198, 199, 200, 201, 202, 203 Squamous cell carcinoma Although many malignant neoplasms may affect the oral cavity, squamous cell carcinoma is by far the most common. It may develop in a previous red or white mucosal lesion, or may appear *ab initio* with no obvious premalignant stage. The lesion shown in **197**, associated with tobacco chewing, eventually developed into the exophitic carcinoma shown in **198**, in spite of a relatively reassuring biopsy report on the original lesion. **199** shows a carcinoma of the lateral margin of the tongue, with no known precursor lesion, developing as an irregular red and white patch

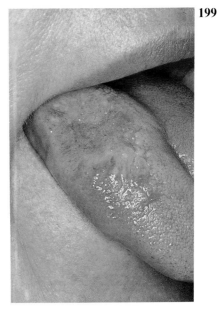

199

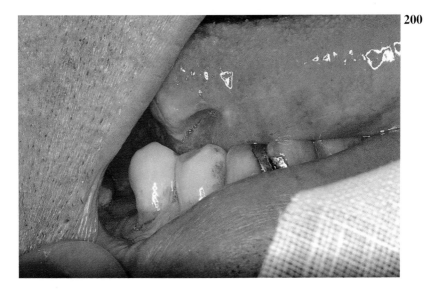

200

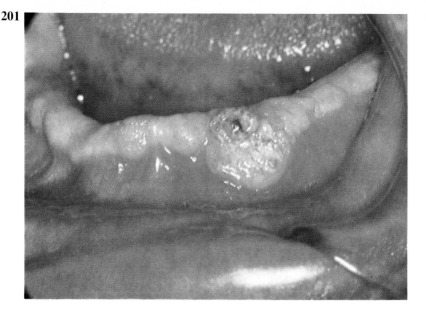

with minimal ulceration, while that in **200** presents as an ulcer with raised, indurated margins. Others may present as apparently innocuous white patches (**201**) or nodules (**202**). Pain is an inconstant symptom and, in a few patients, widespread proliferative lesions may occur with minimal complaint (**203**).

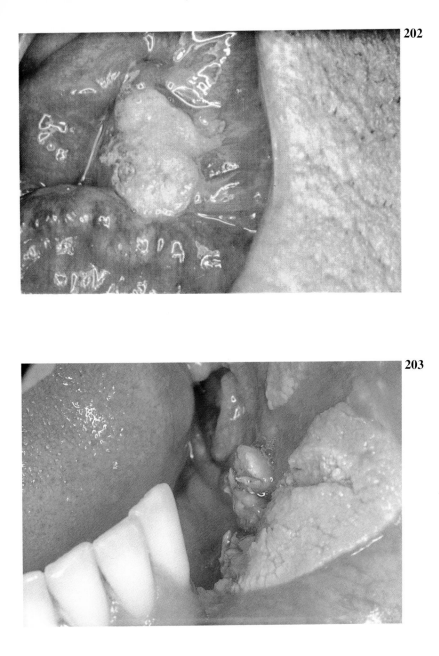

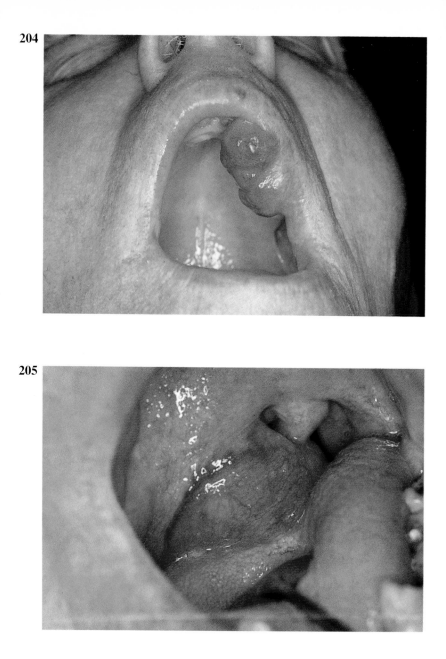

204,205,206,207,208 Other malignant lesions Other malignant lesions may occur either primarily in the oral soft tissues, as part of a more generalized process or by extension from a bony origin. These three examples illustrate each category. The appearances are characteristic but by no means diagnostic: definitive diagnosis is entirely by histological study of biopsy material. **204** shows an adenocystic carcinoma originating in the upper lip, **205** a pharyngeal lesion in generalized non Hodgkins lymphoma, while **206** shows an aggressive angiosarcoma spreading into the oral cavity from the mandible. Very occasionally the oral cavity may be involved in direct

206

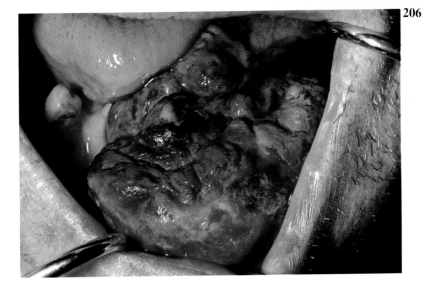

207

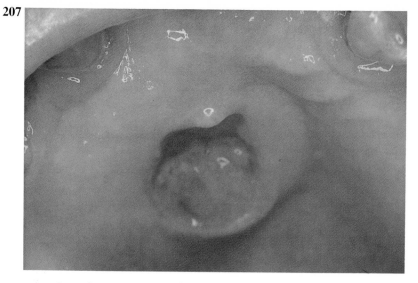

extension of an extraoral neoplasm. **207** shows an intraoral extension of the basal cell carcinoma of the facial skin shown (post operatively) in **208**.

208

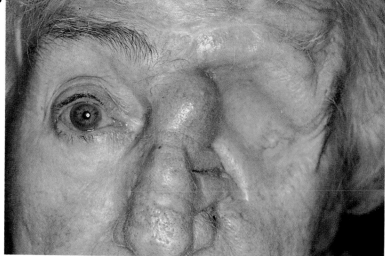

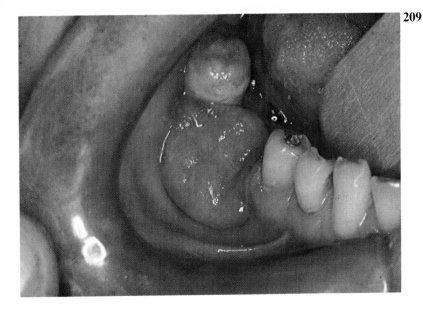

209 Secondary neoplasm This lesion is a secondary neoplasm arising from a primary adenocarcinoma of the oesophagogastric junction. The location of the metastasis — in the socket of a recently extracted tooth — has been described in a number of cases. It is thought possible that there may be direct seeding of the socket by malignant cells derived from the primary neoplasm, free in the oral cavity.

210,211 Malignant melanoma of the palate This malignant melanoma of the palate (**210**) was described in the first edition of this atlas as resembling caviar spread on the palate. Clearly this is a good descriptive term. The clinical differential diagnosis of melanotic patches that may not show such signs of exuberant overgrowth may be very difficult. Such lesions as benign melanotic naevi (**211**), or even amalgam tattoos in the mucosa, may come under suspicion, particularly when noticed for the first time. The necessity to carry out excisional biopsy on lesions that might be malignant melanomas may make even the decision to biopsy a difficult one.

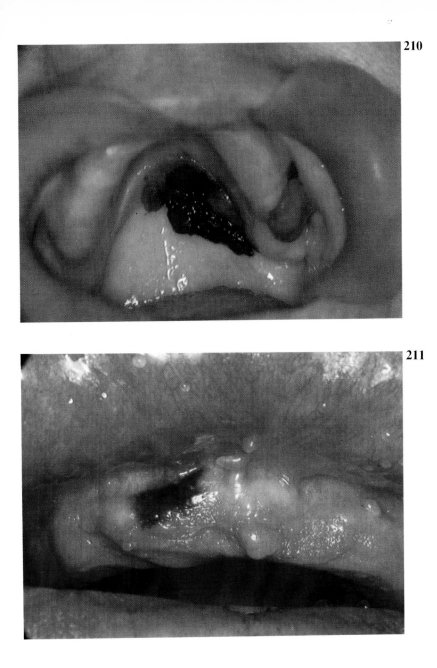

212,213 Mucous cysts These are examples of mucous cysts (or mucoceles). They may occur anywhere on the oral mucosa, but commonly on the lower lip or commissure. They are largely extravasation cysts — the result of the collection of mucous in the soft tissues following the rupture of a mucous gland duct by trauma. The blue colour of the cyst in **212** is characteristic, but in **213** the lesion has a pink colour and could be mistaken, on appearance alone, for a fibro-epithelial polyp. However, the texture on palpation is diagnostic. A less common form of mucous cyst arises by blockage (rather than rupture) of the duct. This is the mucous retention cyst, which has similar clinical features to the extravasation cyst: it is clinically virtually impossible to distinguish them.

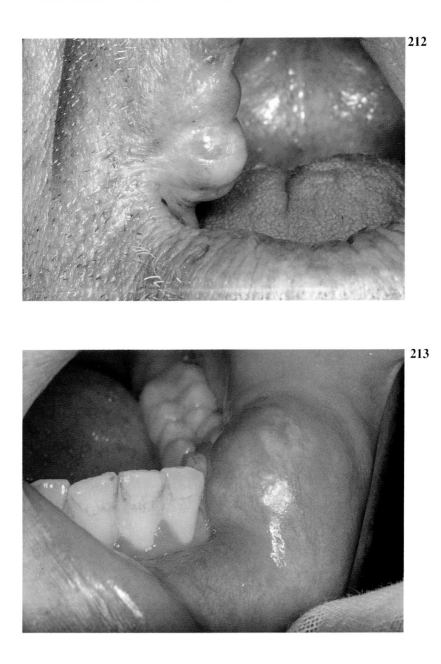

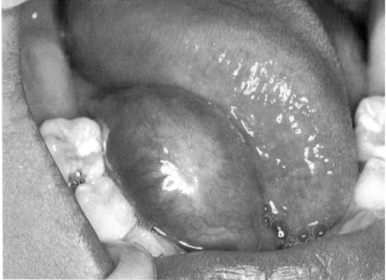

214 Ranula This is a ranula: a cystic lesion of the floor of the mouth. It is a clinical diagnosis: the origin of such a cyst may be either in the major sublingual gland or in sublingually placed minor salivary glands. A very few of these lesions undergo expansion downwards through the tissue spaces of the neck, and may pose a difficult surgical problem: the plunging ranula.

The tongue

The tongue has a special role in oral disease processes because of its specialized epithelial covering, which particularly depends for its integrity on the maintenance of good general health. In a wide range of generalized diseases (particularly anaemias and related conditions), the normal epithelial structure of the tongue is changed, often by loss of the normal papillary structure.

The tongue is also particularly susceptible to trauma: both primary trauma (as, for instance, from a fractured tooth) and secondary damage that might follow (for example) reduced salivary flow.

A few lesions (such as hairy tongue, **229**) are restricted entirely to the tongue since they completely depend on abnormalities in the tongue's unique surface structure.

215 Tongue-tie Shown is the most common developmental abnormality of the tongue, tongue-tie, which may result from either a short lingual frenum, or one that extends unusually well forward to the tip of the tongue. It generally causes no trouble, although the frenum can become ulcerated with trauma.

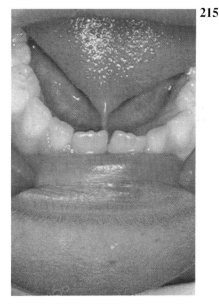

215

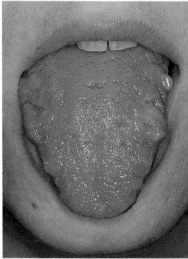

216 Crenated tongue Fissures and unusual tongue morphology, as in this crenated (scalloped) tongue, often cause concern when first noticed by the patient. On the whole, however, except in chronic infections of long standing (as, for example, in **96**) and a very few conditions that lead to fibrotic changes, the basic fissure pattern and general morphology of the tongue remains unchanged through life. It is true, however, that superficial infections or other mucosal abnormalities may appear initially in the depths of fissures and give the impression of causing the fissures to occur.

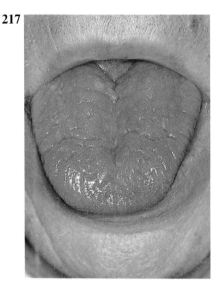

217,218,219 Depapillation of the tongue The maintenance of the complex surface structure of the tongue depends on many factors: including, in particular, the presence of a normal blood picture. Generalized loss of the filiform papillae may occur in anaemias and many other related haematological conditions. The loss of the fililform papillae seems to be an important feature leading to the sore tongue in acute atrophic candidiasis. The lateral margin of the tongue is particularly susceptible to irritation by trauma in these circumstances (**218**). It can,

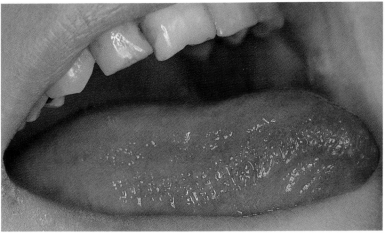

however, be difficult to distinguish clinically between simple trauma, the onset of a more generalized superficial glossitis, and lesions such as those of localized erosive lichen planus (**219**).

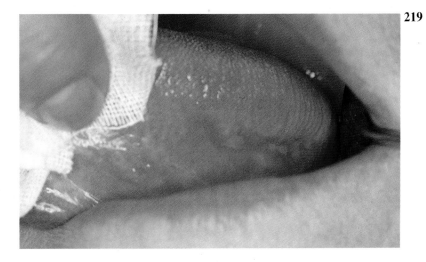

220,221,222,223   Geographic tongue   The patchy depapillation that occurs in geographic tongue is not understood. In this condition the filiform papillae disappear from the surface of the tongue in localized areas. The resultant red patches are characteristically surrounded by a white zone of slightly disrupted epithelium, but this is not invariable. The patches may last for a variable time, then repapillate, to form again later in another site on the tongue. There has been much speculation as to possible relationships between geographic tongue and other conditions — particularly psoriasis — but no firm connection has been convincingly demonstrated. In some patients the lesions may be solitary and effectively static (**223**); these often cause considerable diagnostic confusion.

220

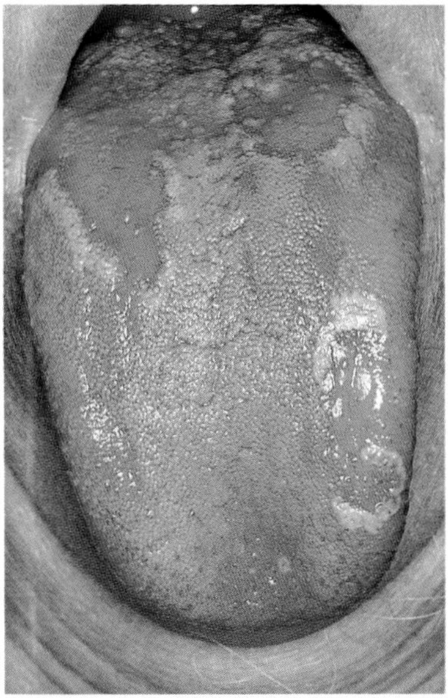

221

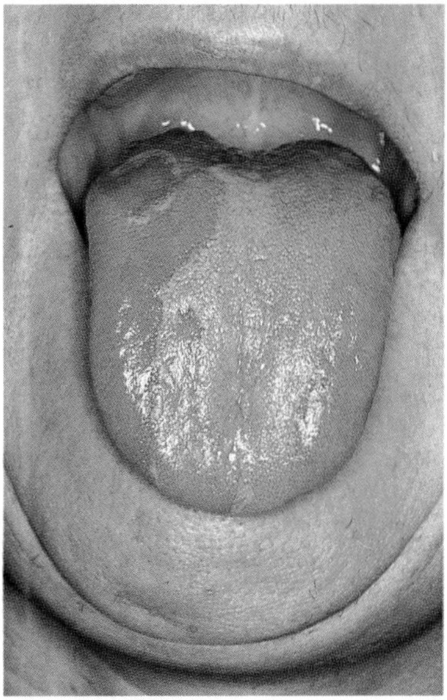

222

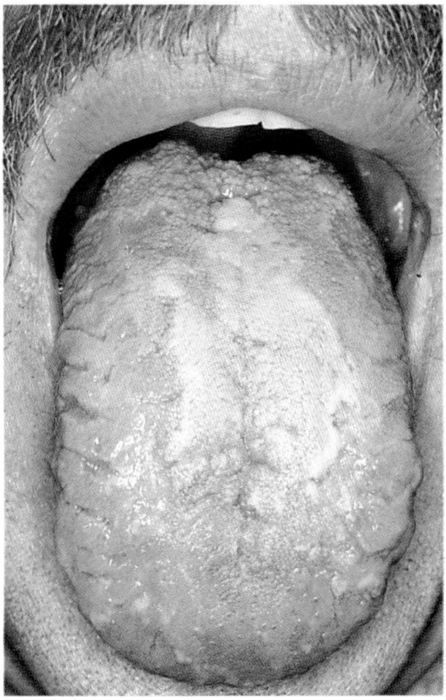

223

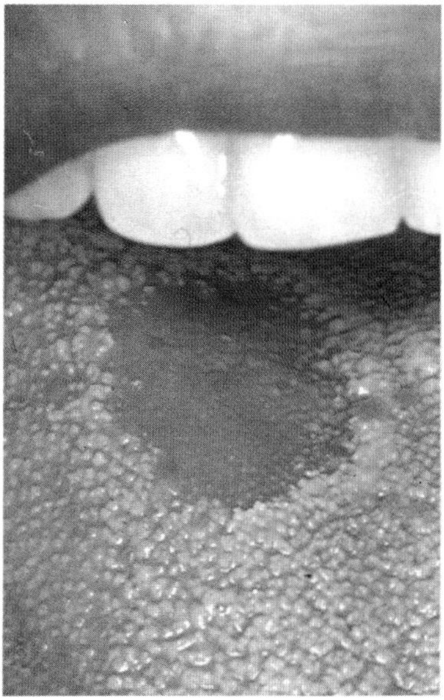

224 Geographic patches with crenated tongue It has been suggested that geographic patches associated with a crenated tongue pattern constitutes a separate entity, but there is no real evidence for this.

225 Lichen planus A somewhat similar appearance to that of geographic tongue may be seen in some keratotic lesions, particularly in lichen planus (**225**). The history and behaviour are, however, quite different.

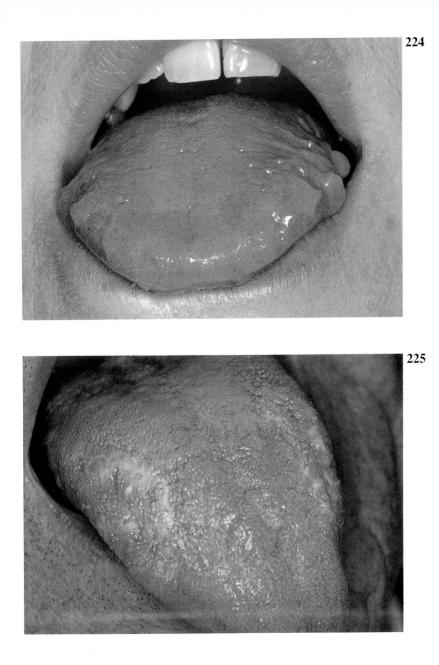

226

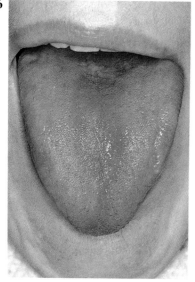

226,227,228 Midline glossitis
Midline glossitis was for long thought to be a developmental defect. It is now known, however, to be associated with chronic candidal infection of the epithelium. There are many patterns, some of which consist of erythematous patches (**226**), some including faint white lesions together with the erythema (**227**) and some that are rather proliferative in appearance (**228**). These lesions are often mistaken for premalignant conditions or even, in the case of the proliferative form, for carcinomas. In fact the premalignant potential is relatively low.

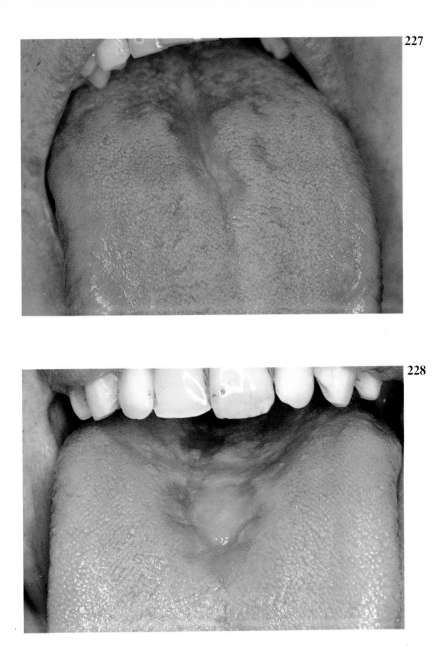

229,230 Hairy tongue Black or brown hairy tongue is a condition in which the filiform papillae elongate to form a "hairy" coating to the tongue. There is no explanation either for the elongation of the papillae or for the colouration that then occurs. Chromogenic bacteria used to be implicated but, in fact, have never been demonstrated. Numerous precipitating factors have been described: antibiotics, antiseptic mouthwashes, excessive tobacco and so on. Some hairy tongues appear without any apparent precipitating factor of any kind.

231 Allergic reaction The tongue is often particularly involved in acute allergic reactions, and may consequently pose a danger to the airway. Here is a swelling, largely confined to half of the tongue, as part of a generalized reaction to penicillin.

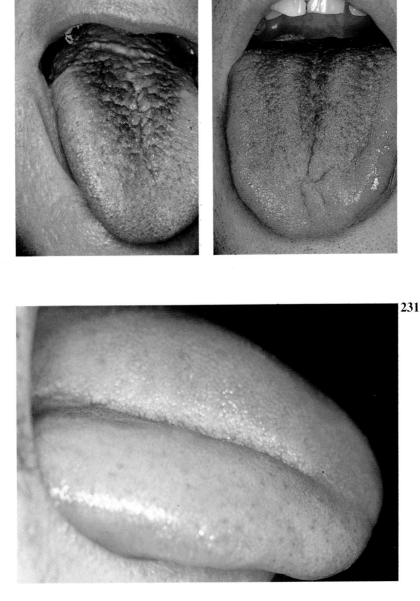

232   Carcinoma of the lateral border of the tongue   Carcinoma of the tongue has been shown earlier (**199,200**). Here is a further example of a carcinoma of the lateral border of the tongue arising in a *Candida leukoplakia*. The diagnosis and management of lesions in this site is of crucial importance: a high proportion of carcinomas of the lateral margin of the tongue have produced cervical metastases at the time of initial diagnosis.

233   Haemangioma   within   the   tongue   The   propensity   of angiomatous lesions to occur in the tongue has also been mentioned. This is a further example of a haemangioma deep within the substance of the tongue and easily capable of misdiagnosis.

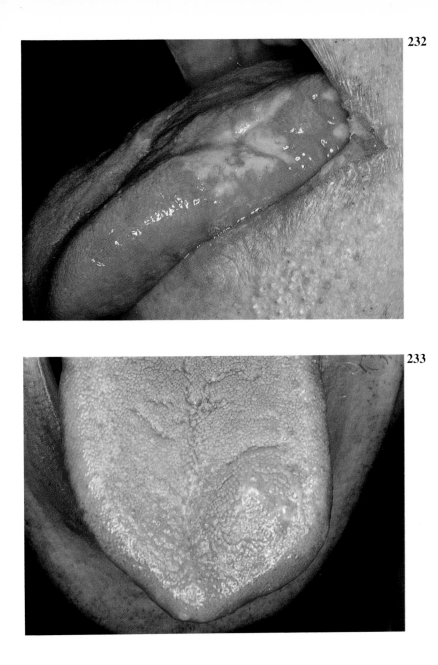

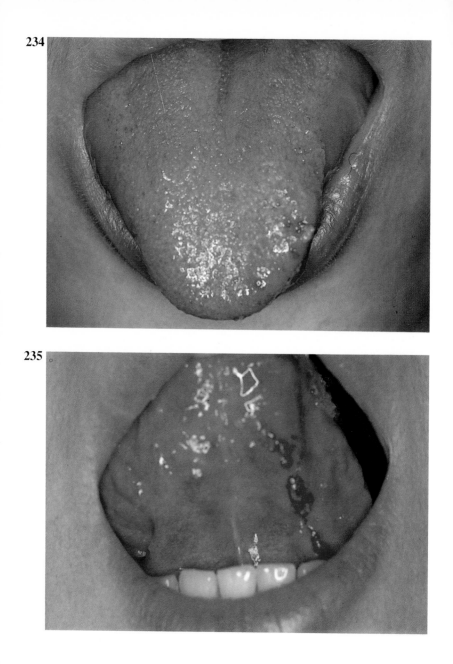

234

235

184

234,235 Angiomatous lesions Other angiomatous lesions of the tongue have elements both of lymphangioma and haemangioma.

236 Atrophy of the tongue This is a well known neurological sign, but one rarely presenting for diagnosis in clinics devoted to orofacial diseases. It is an example of atrophy of the left side of the tongue following a lesion of the hypoglossal nerve.

236

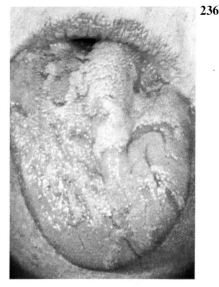

237

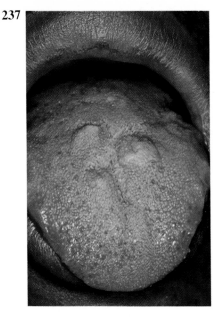

237 von Recklinghausen's disease This is also a well documented but relatively rare condition: the occurrence of multiple neurofibromas of the tongue in von Recklinghausen's disease. This is a genetically determined condition in which the lesions (which are hamartomas rather than true neoplasms) involve the oral mucosa, and particularly the tongue, in a small proportion of cases.

Teeth and gingivae

The teeth do not indicate current disease processes, except in a very few cases: for instance, when decalcification may occur from the introduction of acidic fluids into the mouth from the stomach. They may much more frequently indicate abnormal metabolic states in the patient at the time of tooth formation. It may be possible to assess quite accurately the timing of such events by the resulting dental tissue abnormality. Abnormalities in the shape and eruption pattern of the teeth may have only local significance or may be associated with disorders of skin, bone or other tissues. However, many clinical dental problems are essentially inflammatory in origin, mostly stemming from the progression from caries to pulp involvement to periapical lesion.

The term hypoplasia has two separate meanings in relation to the teeth. It is used as a clinical term to describe a general disturbance of tooth structure. It is also used more specifically to indicate a deficiency in the enamel matrix prior to calcification. It thus distinguishes conditions caused by such a deficiency from those resulting from an imperfect calcification process: hypocalcification. In view of the developmental interrelationship between enamel and dentine, conjoint abnormalities may occur in either of these situations; but this is not always the case. Indeed, most abnormalities may be described as either of enamel or of dentine.

The gingivae, on the contrary, being the site of active metabolic and cellular activity, may quite rapidly reflect generalized disease processes. However, the resultant changes are specific in only a few cases: most gingival responses to generalized disease can be explained in terms of modified (usually exaggerated) degrees of inflammatory change.

238,239 Irregular teeth eruption   Although in some unusual cases disturbance of the eruption pattern of the teeth may be associated with generalized abnormalities — for example, of bone growth — by far the most common causes of irregular eruption are local and dependant on such factors as disproportionate tooth size compared with skeletal size. **238** shows a typical example of this. In **239** a similar situation is complicated by the lack of exfoliation of the deciduous dentition. This probably results from the absence of the normal processes of resorption, which are stimulated by the eruption of the permanent dentition.

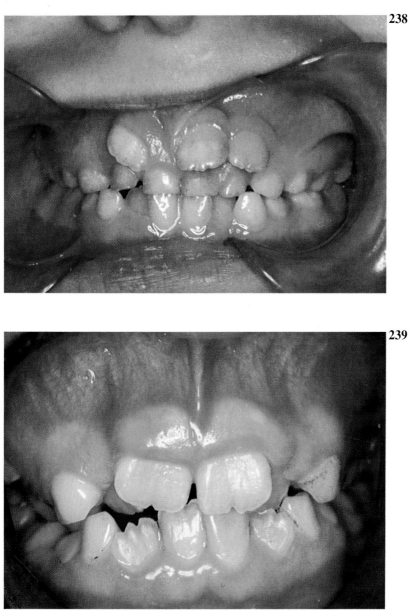

238

239

240,241 Supernumerary teeth The presence of supernumerary teeth may also cause irregularity in the eruption pattern, as in **240**. The midline of the upper incisor region is the most common site of such isolated supernumerary teeth (often termed mesiodens). In **241** the presence of such a tooth has led to the delayed eruption of both permanent central incisors.

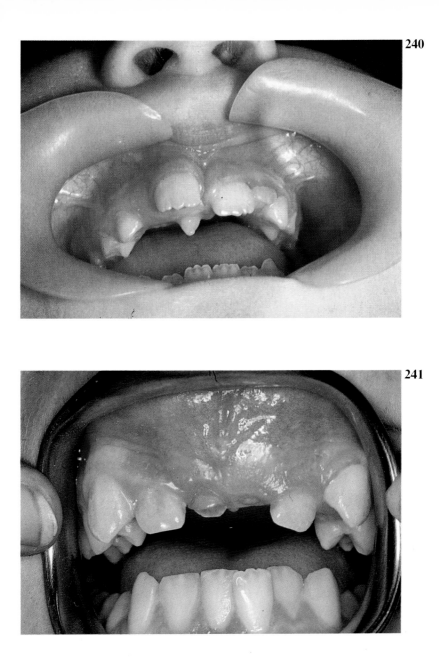

242 Cyst of eruption In this patient the delayed eruption of the right permanent incisor has led to the formation of a so called cyst of eruption. This is a common occurrence, even in teeth that are not particularly late in erupting, and can almost be counted a normal finding unless it remains present for a protracted time.

243 Dentigerous cyst Shown here is a dentigerous cyst associated with the unerupted first premolar. Such lesions may be entirely intrabony or, as in this case, may partially expand into the mouth, thus to some extent resembling a more extensive cyst of eruption.

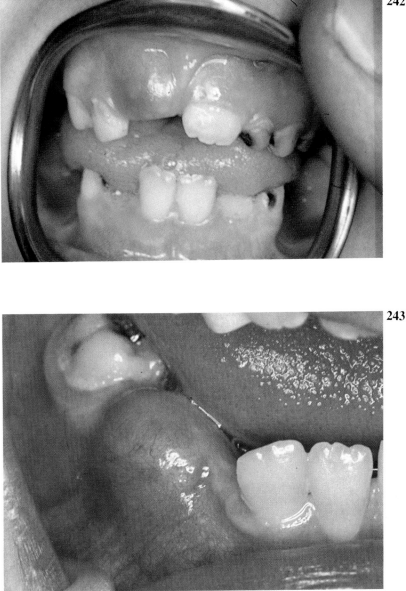

244,245 Connation These are two examples of connation, a term used to imply the growing together of two units. This may be the result of the fusion of the normal developing tooth germ with a supernumerary germ (fusion). Alternatively, it may in some instances result from the development and partial separation of two teeth from a single tooth germ (gemination). It occurs in both the deciduous and permanent dentitions, and there is often a genetic basis to the condition.

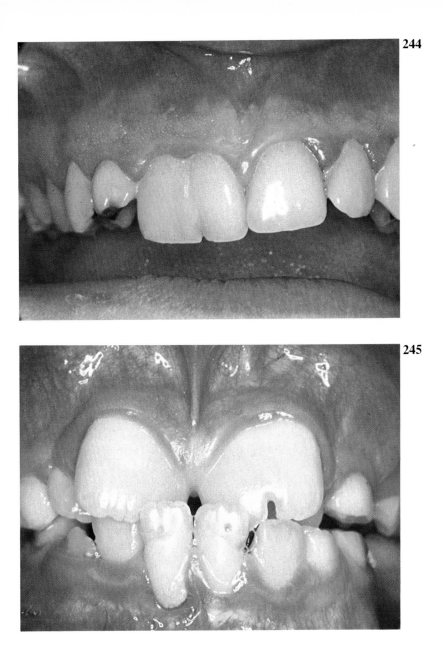

246 Rampant caries Rampant caries in a young patient. In these circumstances the carious process may be too fast to allow the defence reactions of the dentine and pulp to occur. There may therefore be early pulp involvement.

247 Gross caries Gross caries in an adult in whom the initial tooth substance loss was due to exposure to industrial acids.

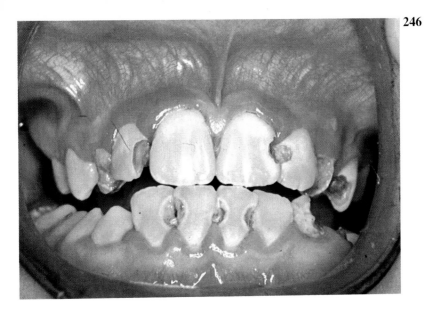

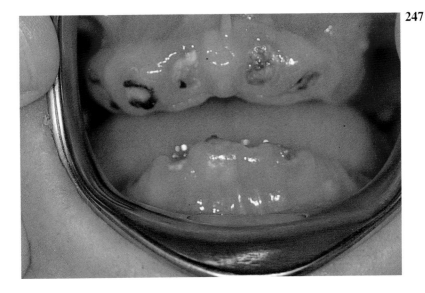

248

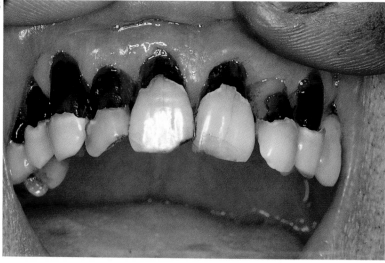

249

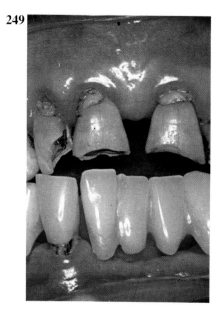

248 Cervical caries Cervical caries with heavy tobacco staining of the lesions. On the whole, cervical caries is slowly progressive.

249 Cervical caries associated with xerostomia Cervical caries in a patient with xerostomia. This is a common finding in patients with Sjögren's syndrome and similar conditions, and also following radiotherapy to the head and neck. In this patient the shiny atrophic mucosa seen in xerostomia is also well shown.

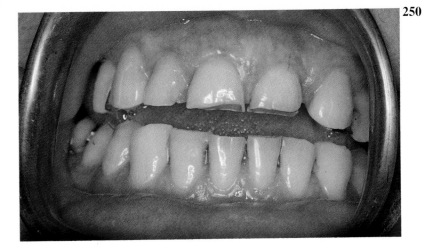

250 Attrition of teeth Attrition — the wear caused by tooth to tooth contact — is, to some extent, a physiological process. However, in patients such as the one shown here with occlusal problems, the enamel loss may become significant and may lead to exposure of considerable amounts of dentine.

251 Attrition of teeth Attrition may also become a problem in those patients with abnormalities either of tooth morphology or structure. This is an adult patient with attrition complicating microdontia. These are not deciduous teeth, but abnormally small permanent teeth.

252 Abrasion of teeth Abrasion is the term used to describe tooth substance loss due to trauma from an external source: the most common by far being the toothbrush. This is an example of severe tooth brush abrasion. Two teeth have been so deeply abraded that the crowns have broken off. This is a slow procedure and, as a result, there is little pain and the dentino-pulpal reactions protect the remaining tooth and pulp.

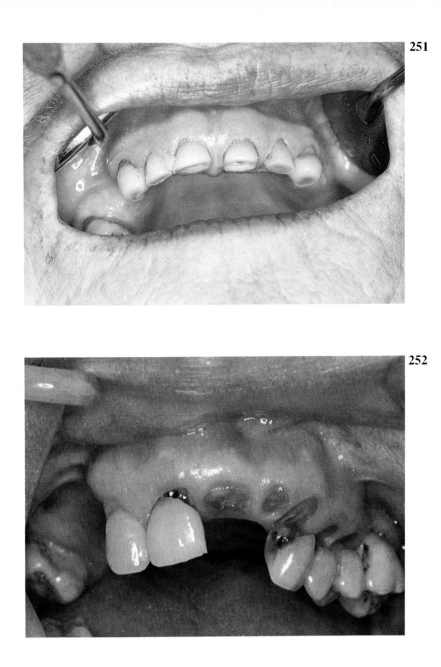

251

252

253 Dietary tooth erosion Acid erosion of tooth substance used to be predominantly the result of industrial activity; **247** has demonstrated the possible end result of this. However, dietary habits have now become a significant factor in the aetiology of acid erosion. This female patient had taken a large number of grapefruit daily as part of a "healthy" diet. She had also used her toothbrush vigorously. The resulting loss of tooth substance is shown. Most cases of dietary tooth erosion are a result of acid erosion coupled with abrasion and/or attrition.

254 Tooth erosion from vomiting These are the palatal surfaces of the upper anterior teeth of a young female patient affected by bulimia nervosa with vomiting. The loss of tooth substance is evident.

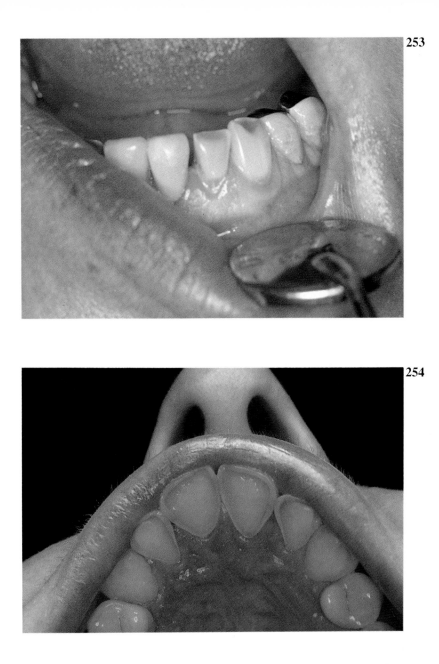

255 Simple trauma to the upper incisors This illustrates simple trauma to the upper incisors in a young patient — a very common injury. In general, fractures of this kind do not involve the pulp, and (although they may initially be painful and require treatment) they do not result in loss of vitality.

256 Extensive tooth fracture This is a more extensive fracture involving the pulp. Pulp death has occurred, followed by discolouration of the tooth.

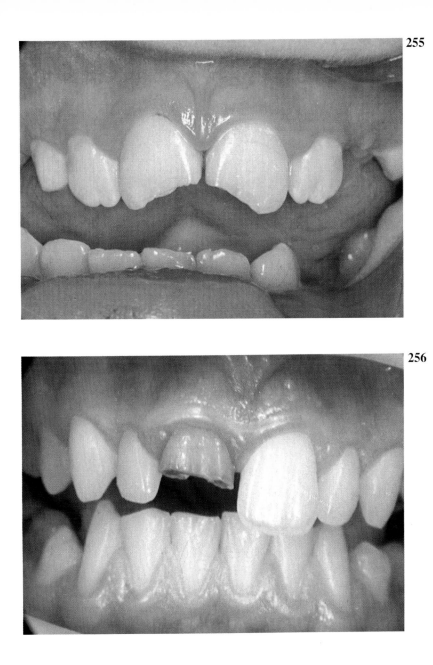

257 Pulp death Trauma to these two central incisors, although resulting in only very minor fractures of the enamel, has resulted in pulp death. The resultant discolouration is usually attributed to the aspiration of blood pigments into the dentinal tubules.

258 Internal idiopathic resorption This is internal idiopathic resorption (pink spot). Generally following evident trauma (as in this case), the pink colour represents pulp tissue visible through the thinned wall of the tooth. The degree of resorption may be extensive and, in a few cases, may lead to perforation.

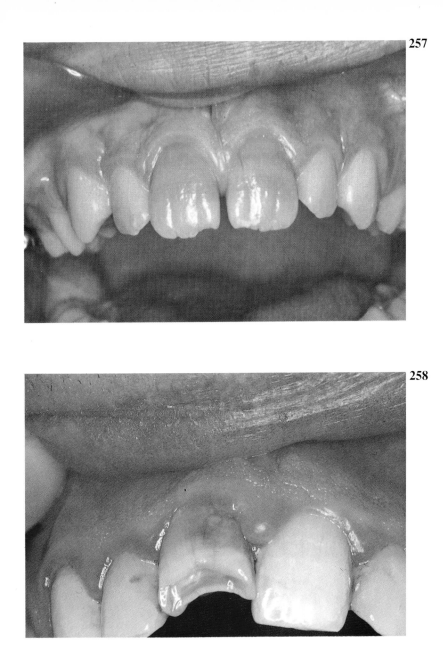

259 Rickets   Illustrated here is severe disturbance of the formation of both enamel and dentine in rickets. This, as here, is classically associated with an anterior open bite resulting from abnormal jaw development.

260 Hypoplasia   This is a much more restricted form of hypoplasia in a patient with coeliac disease. The disturbance in calcium metabolism, occurring with the intake of gluten at weaning, is reflected in the hypoplastic band on the lower central incisors. This is an example of the so called chronological hypoplasia.

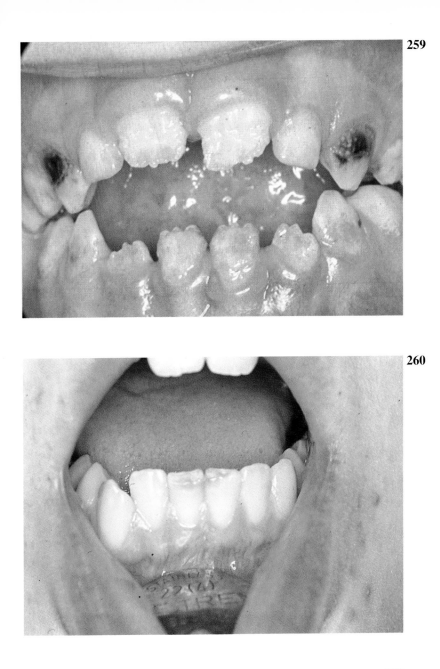

261

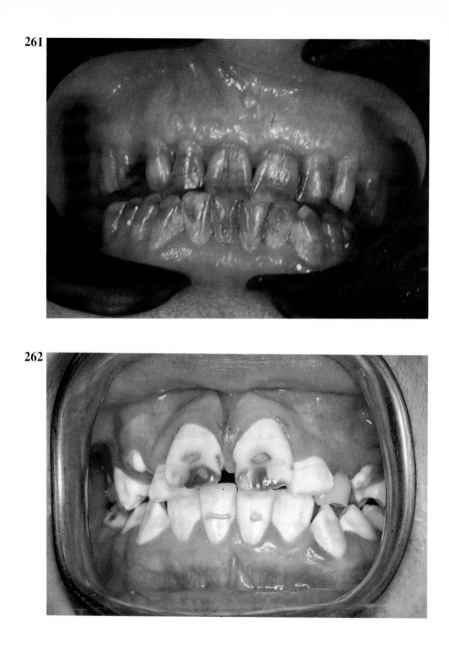

262

261,262 Enamel hypoplasia This (**261**) is a gross example of enamel hypoplasia associated with a high fluoride intake. Most patients with fluorosis have mottled, rather than uniformly stained, teeth (**262**). The origin of the brown pigmentation is still not known.

263 Morphological hypoplasia These teeth are small and abnormally formed: hypoplastic in the morphological sense of that term. This is a developmental abnormality; the resemblance to the teeth in congenital syphilis shown in **269, 270** is not very close. The lack of suppression of the central tubercles is a diagnostic indicator against a syphilitic origin for this hypoplasia.

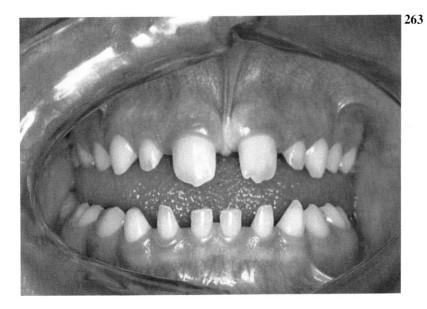

263

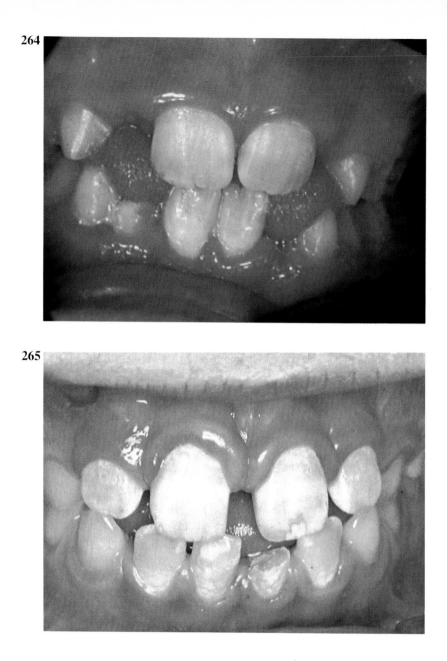

264,265,266   Hypocalcification type of amelogenesis imperfecta These show the hypocalcification type of amelogenesis imperfecta. The opaque white enamel is characteristic. The pattern shown in **266** results in the so called "snow capped" teeth.

266

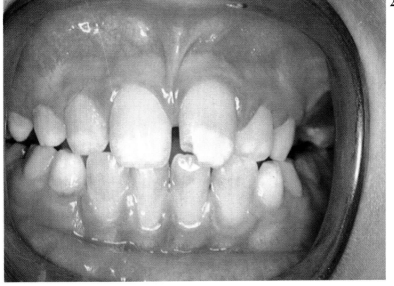

267 Hypocalcification type of amelogenesis imperfecta This is a further example of the hypocalcification form of amelogenesis imperfecta where caries has occurred in an uncontrolled way. This family included a mother and two daughters with essentially the same problem.

268 Hypoplastic type of amelogenesis imperfecta Shown is the hypoplastic type of amelogenesis imperfecta. The remaining enamel is fully calcified but, because of its deficient bulk, has been worn away from the affected teeth.

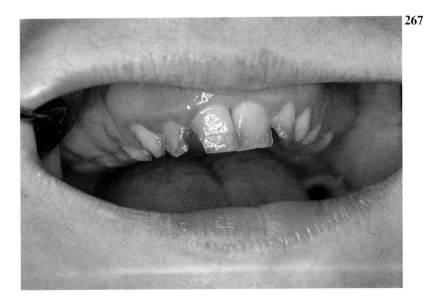

267

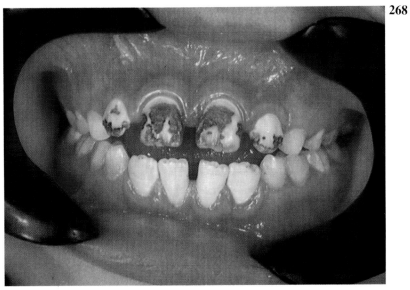

268

269,270 Hutchinson's incisors A classical cause of enamel hypoplasia is seen in the Hutchinson's incisors of congenital syphilis, in which there is modification of the shape of the teeth due to the growth of the spirochaetes in the tooth germ itself. The rounded shape of the maxillary incisors shown in **269** is often described, but a much more dramatic presentation is shown in **270**, where there are much more marked changes in the enamel and in the morphology of the teeth. The suppression of the central tubercle of the tooth with resultant notching of the incisal edge is said to be characteristic.

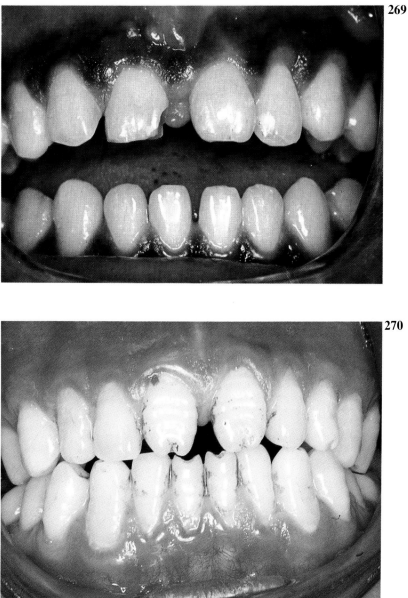

269

270

271,272 Dentinogenesis imperfecta   This is dentinogenesis imperfecta of the deciduous (**272**) and permanent (**271**) dentitions. A clinical term used to describe this genetic abnormality is hereditary opalescent dentine. The teeth have various colours: the bluish tinge shown in **271** is that most commonly described. This is a condition usually entirely confined to the dentine, although something very like it may occur in patients with osteogenesis imperfecta, presumably as a result of a generalized mesodermal calcification defect. Although the enamel is not structurally affected, it may become detached from the dentine because of weakness at the dentino-enamel junction. The pulp chambers are often filled by the growth of abnormal dentine.

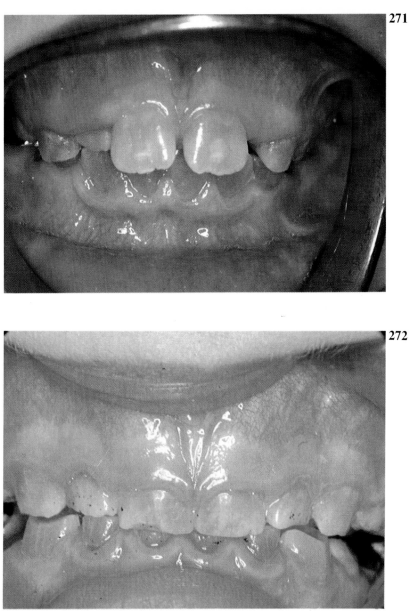

271

272

273 Tetracycline staining   This is a remarkably good illustration of the effect of tetracyclines in marking calcifying tissues at the time of administration. Tetracyclines should not be used in children under 12 years or pregnant women because of this problem. The ability of this group of antibiotics to clearly mark the state of development of teeth and bone has led to their use in many experimental procedures.

274 Tetracycline staining   Shown is a clinical picture of tetracycline staining, combined with hypoplastic changes resulting from the persistent generalized infective conditions for which the antibiotic had been given. A single tooth has been restored.

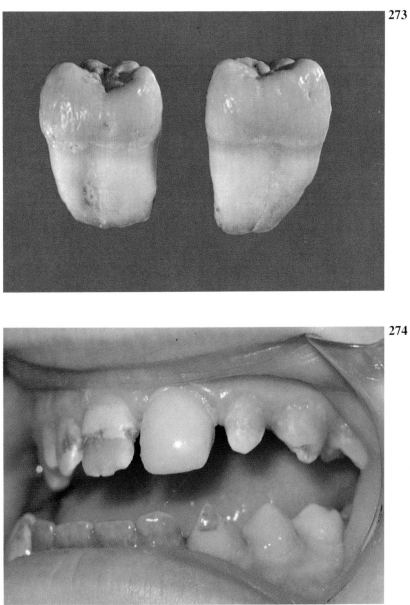

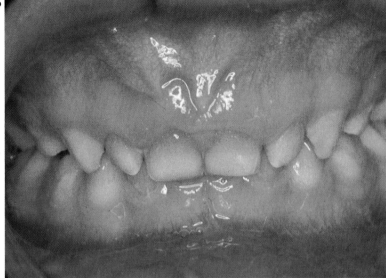

275 Tetracycline staining   This illustrates tetracycline staining in the deciduous dentition following administration to the mother during pregnancy.

276,277 Extrinsic staining of teeth   These illustrate the tooth staining that may occur in the deciduous (**277**) and permanent (**276**) dentitions in conditions of poor oral hygiene. The exact causative factor for the colouration in this extrinsic staining is not known. In **276** there is also a gross occlusal abnormality affecting the anterior teeth.

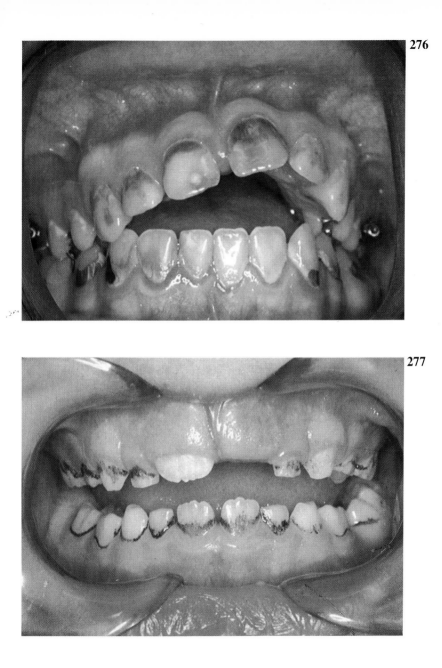

276

277

278 Alveolar sinus This is a sinus arising from a chronic periapical abscess at the apex of a deciduous incisor. Such gum boils are very common. At the time of the illustration the sinus is not discharging pus; this tends to be an intermittent process.

279 Discharging sinus This is a similar (but discharging) sinus, arising from a periapical infection on the lateral incisor. Such a sinus may be present for a long time with relatively minor discomfort to the patient.

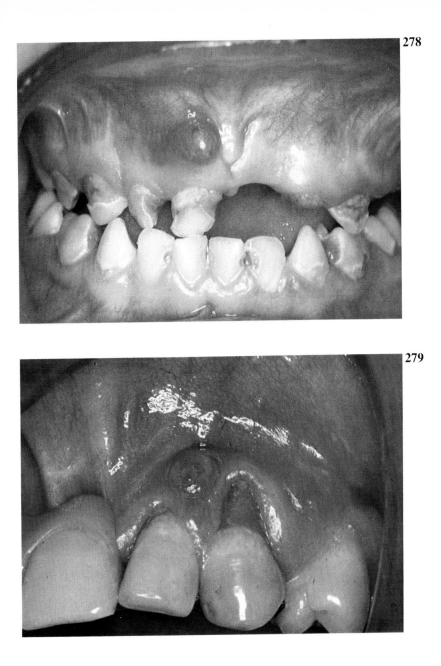

280 Periapical abscess This is a more acute periapical abscess presenting in the buccal sulcus. It may occur as an acute exacerbation of a previous chronic abscess or as the first presentation of the periapical infection. At this point facial swelling, such as that illustrated earlier (**3,4**), may begin.

281 Developing sinus At this stage the appearance of the mucosal lesion may be misleading: this shows a developing sinus with a haemorrhagic appearance, which is not uncommon.

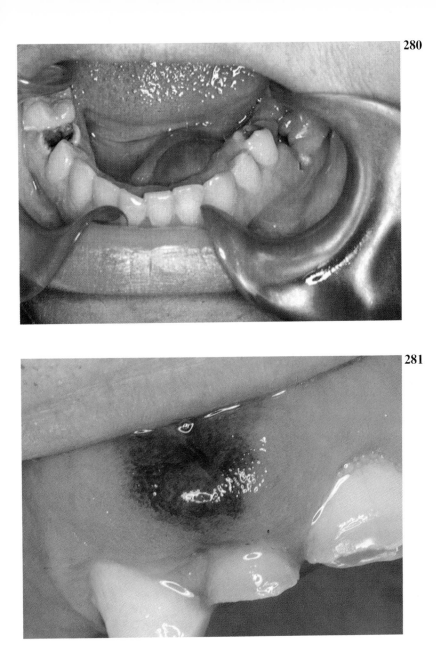

282 Chronic sinus   This chronic sinus has become established, the surrounding mucosa presents a relatively uninflamed appearance, and the lesion could be mistaken for a polyp or epulis.

283 Palatally pointing abscess   This is a palatally pointing abscess resulting from an infection on the upper left lateral incisor. Because of the anatomy in the area, palatal collection of pus from this tooth is not uncommon. The palatal mucosa is very dense, and the pus may track posteriorly under the soft tissues, to point intraorally in a less dense area at the junction of the hard and soft palates.

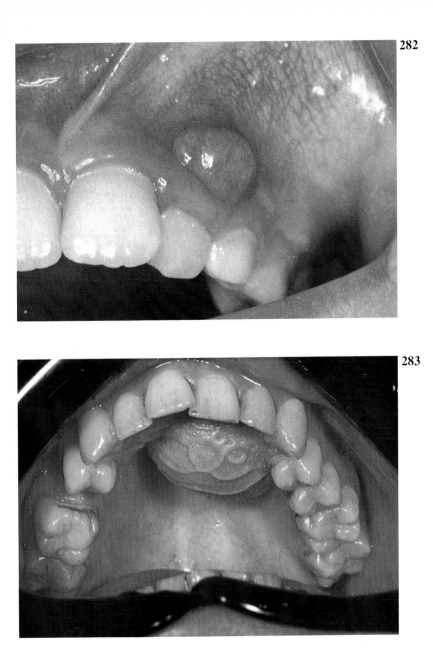

284 Lingually pointing abscess Shown here is a further example of an abscess pointing in a fairly unusual site. The abscess, associated with the lower left first molar, is pointing lingually.

285 Osteomyelitis Osteomyelitis following tooth extraction is a very rare complication in the healthy patient, although a localized osteitis ("dry socket") is common. The multiple sinuses discharging pus are characteristic of the condition. The predominating organism involved is *Staph. aureus*. An active osteomyelitis such as this is likely to occur only in patients with chronic debilitating diseases, diabetes, haematological abnormalities, or other conditions that might result in a depression of the body's defences.

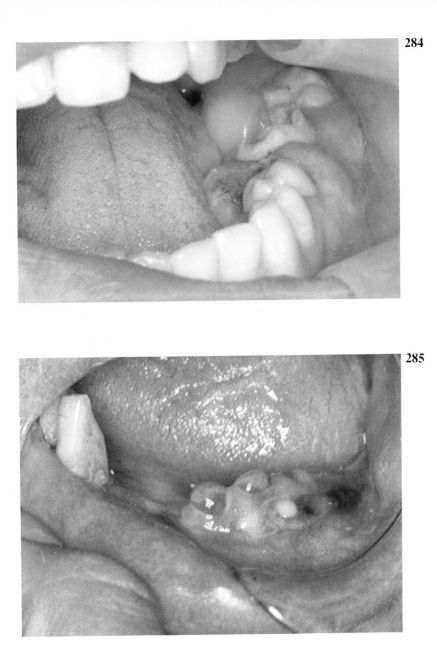

286 Sequestration of necrotic bone The sequestration of necrotic bone is a feature of osteomyelitis, but the picture has been greatly modified in the vast majority of contemporary patients by adequate antibiotic therapy. This patient was in an extremely debilitated condition with a very low haemoglobin level. This form of sequestration, in which the necrotic alveolar bone separates from the basal bone, was a well recognized entity in pre-antibiotic days (alveolar osteomyelitis).

287 Alveolar osteomyelitis This is a dentate patient with alveolar osteomyelitis following agranulocytosis resulting from an adverse reaction to drug therapy. Again, this is a very rare condition.

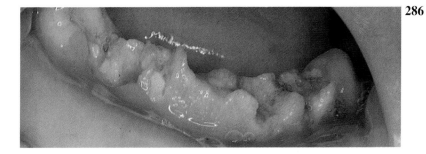

286

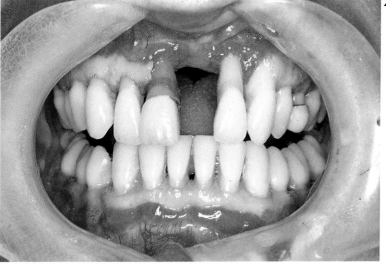

287

288   Chronic osteomyelitis   A further classic presentation: chronic osteomyelitis with a marked proliferative reaction of the periosteum and occasional sequestration of necrotic bone fragments.

289   Chronic osteomyelitis of the mandible   A radiograph of chronic osteomyelitis of the mandible, with patchy decalcification centrally and the laying down of subperiosteal new bone.

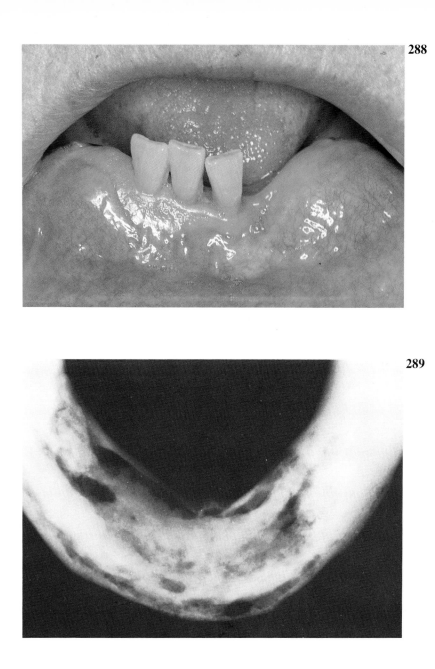

290,291,292 Osteoradionecrosis Osteoradionecrosis is the result of the loss of blood supply to the bone, coupled with deficiency in the repair response of the osteocytes — both brought about as a side effect of radiotherapy. The radiograph shows patchy bone loss. This condition is particularly likely to occur if teeth have to be removed from an irradiated area of the jaws: as shown in **292**, where a tooth has been extracted following radiation. Forward planning should take account of this possibility.

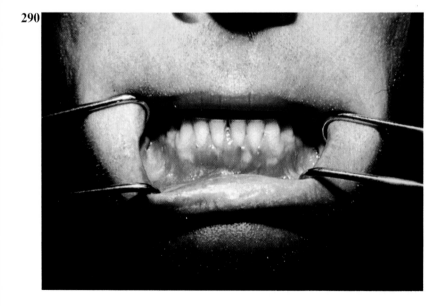

290

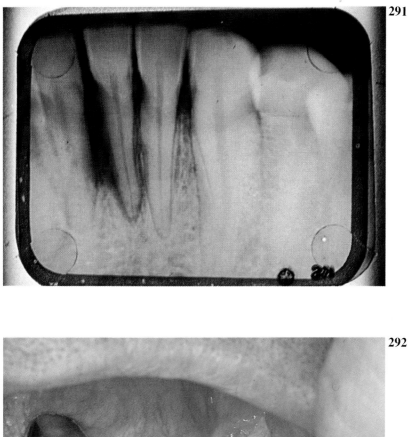

291

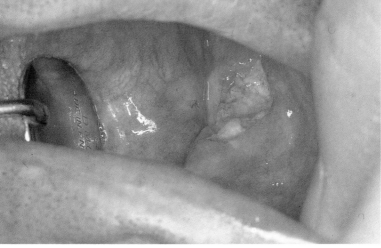

292

293,294 Periapical cyst Periapical cysts may be entirely intrabony and so result in no clinically recognizable expansion of the bone. However, this smooth, rounded lesion, with a bluish colour resulting from thinning of the expanded bony covering, has the quite characteristic appearance of such a cyst. The tooth involved here, the upper lateral incisor, is involved in a high proportion of periapical cysts, presumably because of the high incidence of non vital teeth resulting from palatal invagination and subsequent pulp death. In many cases — but not here — discolouration may give a clue to the non vital tooth of origin of the cyst. The buccal expansion of the thin bony covering is seen in the radiograph.

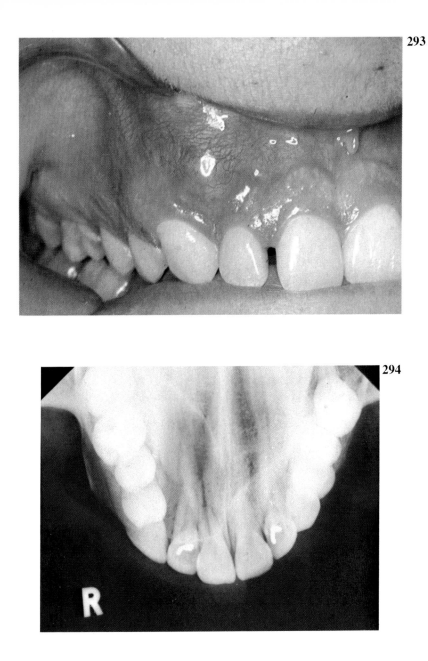

295　Residual dental cyst　This is a residual dental cyst: the tooth that was its origin has been lost (probably extracted), but the periapical cystic lesion has been left behind and has expanded both within the bone and intraorally. The gross dental neglect gives some idea of why such an evident abnormality could have been ignored until this stage of development.

296　Odontogenic　cyst　This　radiograph　demonstrates　the characteristics of a non infected odontogenic cyst. The radiolucent lesion is surrounded by a narrow radio-opaque margin, representing the response of the osteogenic mechanism to the slow and non aggressive expansion of the lesion.

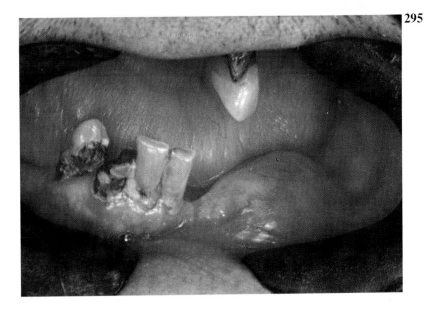

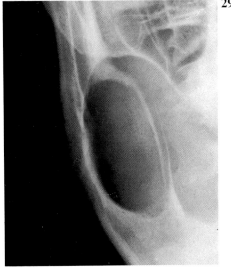

297 Odontogenic keratocyst This is an odontogenic keratocyst of the right maxilla. The site is not the most common — the angle of the mandible is most often involved. This cyst has perforated the buccal bone and the keratin-containing contents are being extruded into the oral cavity. This is rarely seen in mandibular keratocysts. A keratocyst is far more likely to recur and to cause long-term problems than is a simple odontogenic cyst.

298 Soft tissue cyst Although bearing a considerable resemblance to the periapical cyst shown in **293**, this bluish swelling above the upper right lateral incisor is, in fact, a developmental soft tissue cyst. There was no bony involvement and, hence, no radiographic change.

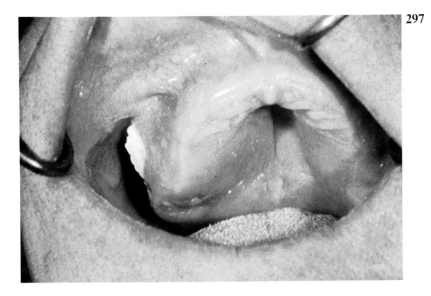

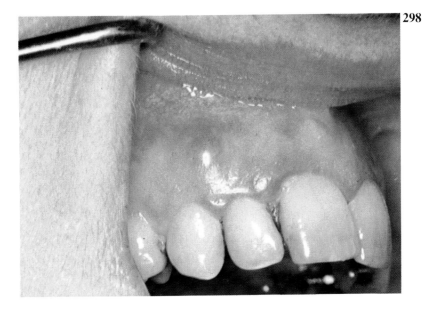

299,300,301 Midline palatal cysts The midline swelling of the palate (**299**) is due to the presence of a developmental cyst. Midline palatal cysts such as this may occur in or at the opening of the incisive canal or, as in this case, posterior to it. The similar lesion shown in **300** is almost entirely intrabony and is visible only as a blue, soft area in the midline of the palate with no soft tissue expansion. However, the radiograph (**301**) shows it to be a quite extensive intrabony lesion.

299

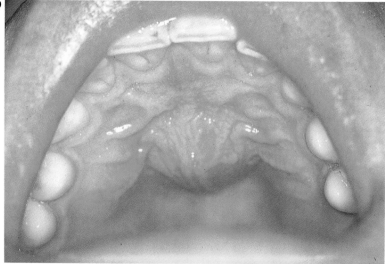

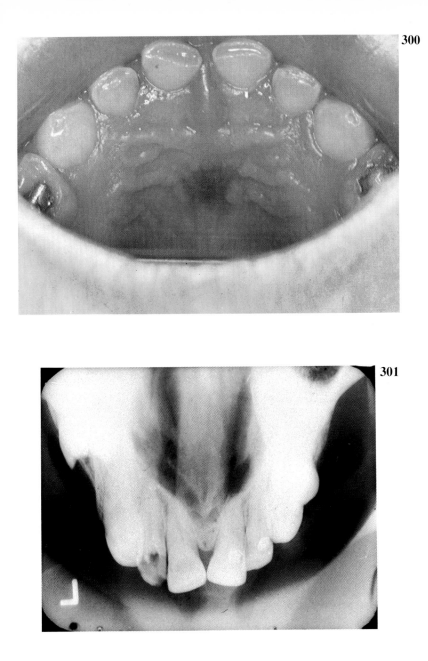

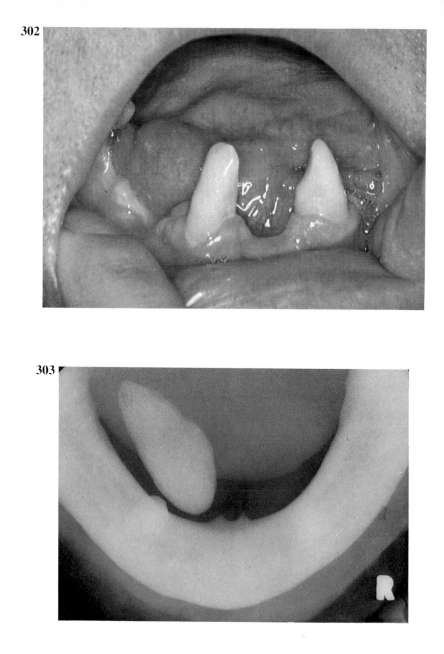

302,303 Submandibular calculus The texture of a swelling such as this (**302**), due to obstruction of the submandibular duct by a calculus, may vary on palpation from soft and cystic to firm or even hard, depending on the size of the calculus, the degree of fibrosis and the presence or otherwise of cystic dilatation of the duct behind the calculus. In this case the calculus was large, as is seen in the radiograph (**303**), and there was little cystic dilatation of the duct. The swelling, therefore, presented as a hard mass.

304 Pulp polyp This is a pulp polyp, the result of chronic hyperplastic pulpitis. It occurs in deciduous and first permanent molars in which the pulp has been widely exposed by gross caries. It consists of granulation tissue derived from the pulp, and is thought to be epithelialized by the implantation and growth of free epithelial cells from the saliva.

304

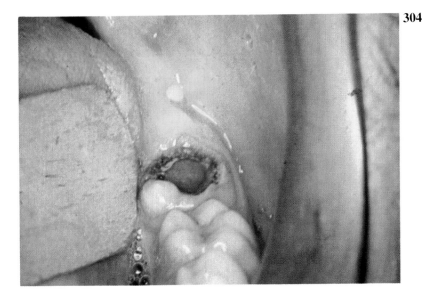

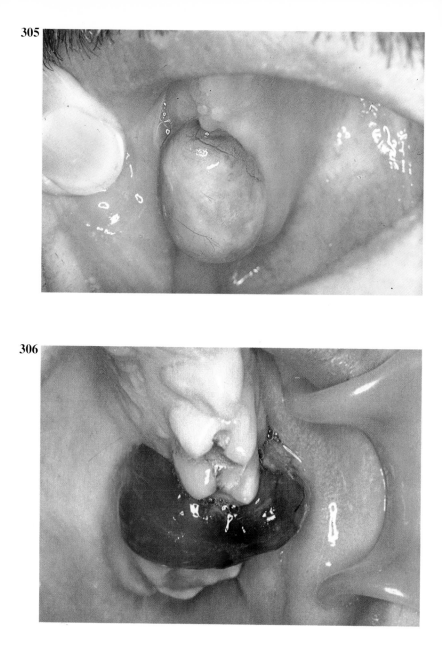

305

306

248

305,306 Prolapsed antral lining A prolapsed antral lining, following the establishment of an oro-antral fistula after the extraction of an upper molar tooth, is shown in **305**. The establishment of such a fistula is not uncommon, but most heal without complications such as this. **306** shows a similar prolapsed antral lining in which an antral polyp is incorporated and into which haemorrhage has occurred.

307 Normal gingivae This is the illustration of normal gingivae shown in the first edition of this atlas. It is, indeed, an excellent picture of uninflamed gingivae — but whether it is as typical as it is normal is another matter: very few individuals have gingivae so free from signs of early periodontal disease.

307

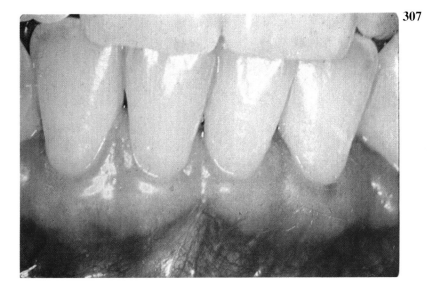

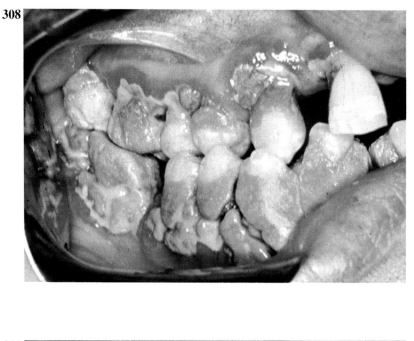

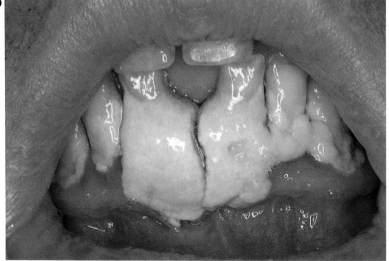

308,309   Extreme oral neglect   In complete contrast to the previous illustration, these are two examples of extreme oral neglect, which is still seen from time to time today in spite of the generally raised level of oral awareness. There is gross deposition of calculus and plaque, and the condition of the periodontal tissues reflects this.

310   Chronic periodontal disease   The oral hygiene of this patient is less deficient than shown in **308** and **309**. Nonetheless, there is marked deposition of plaque and calculus, which has led to chronic periodontal disease and marked distortion of the normal gingival architecture.

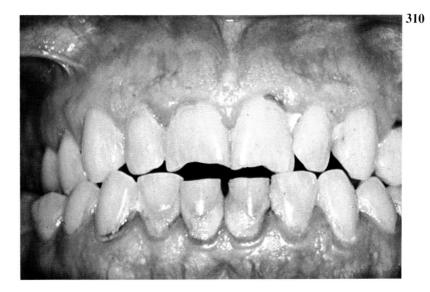

310

311 Severe gingival recession In the previous edition of this atlas this illustration was described as of severe gingival recession that might be an accompaniment of age even in the absence of inflammation. This reflected the viewpoint of the time, but it is now thought that gingival recession of this kind is always associated with some degree of inflammatory change.

312 Marginal gingivitis Marginal gingivitis is shown: the gingival papillae are swollen with a smooth, shiny, red appearance. The plaque deposition (which is largely responsible for the poor gingival condition) is evident.

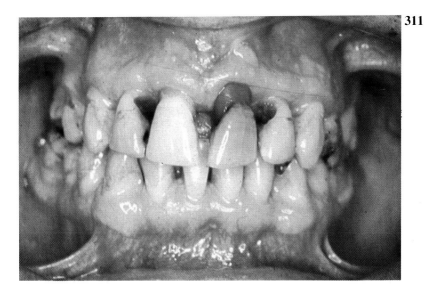

311

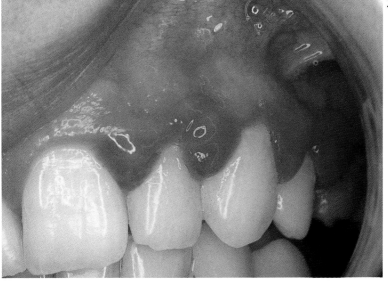

312

313 Gingival recession   This is gingival recession affecting a single tooth. The condition was previously thought to be the result of traumatic occlusion brought about by the position of the tooth, but is now thought to depend entirely on the anatomical factors associated with its malpositioning.

314 Periodontal abscess   A periodontal abscess associated with an upper central incisor. The probe indicates the presence of a deep periodontal pocket that has become acutely infected. Pain and tenderness of the tooth to percussion may lead to confusion with an acute periapical abscess. The differential diagnosis may depend on the fact that the periapical abscess is essentially a lesion associated with a non vital tooth, while the periodontal abscess often occurs in relation to a vital tooth.

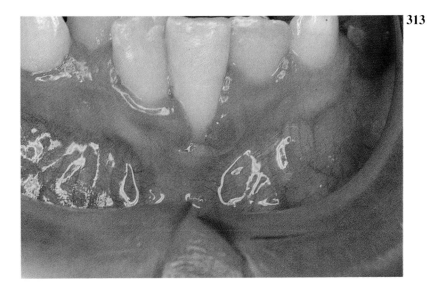

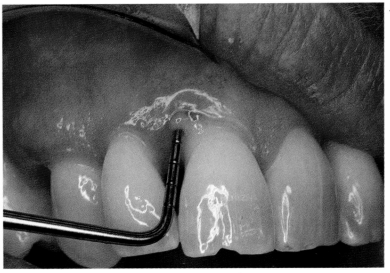

315 Chronic hyperplastic gingivitis This is chronic hyperplastic gingivitis in the upper anterior region that is the result of mouth breathing. It is thus often a consequence of an orthodontic problem. In these circumstances the gingivae are often paler and firmer than in the marginal gingivitis shown in **312**; they are so as the result of an increased fibrous component in the gingivae.

316 Pregnancy gingivitis A hyperplastic gingivitis of a much less fibrous type may occur transiently during periods of hormonal upset: puberty and pregnancy. This is a patient with typical pregnancy gingivitis. There are many views as to why this condition should occur, but it is now generally accepted that it represents an exacerbation of a previously existing chronic gingivitis. It should be emphasized that other conditions, such as desquamative gingivitis, that were previously thought to have an unspecified hormonal basis, are now not thought to have such a connection. Examples of such gingival lesions in lichen planus and pemphigoid have been shown in **160** and **164**.

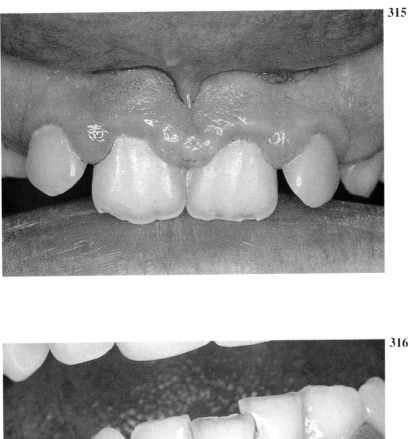

315

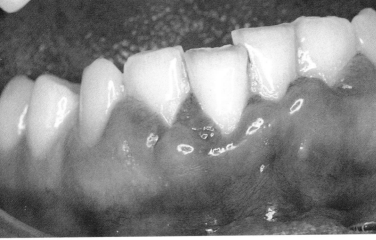

316

317 Pregnancy epulis An occasional feature in pregnancy gingivitis is the growth of a single papilla to form a mass of granulation tissue known as a pregnancy epulis (or pregnancy tumour). The lesion usually regresses completely following the pregnancy.

318,319 Drug induced gingival hyperplasia A hyperplastic gingivitis is a well known side effect of some drug therapy. These are examples of such a response to the anticonvulsant drug phenytoin (**318**) and the immunosuppressant cyclosporin (**319**). Another drug that may cause such a response is the antihypertensive agent nifedipine, which is often given at the same time as cyclosporin to renal transplant patients. In all these cases the gingival response is essentially fibroblastic. It has been suggested that an immaculate oral hygiene regime is sufficient to hold such gingival changes at bay; experience, however, suggests that this is not always a practical possibility.

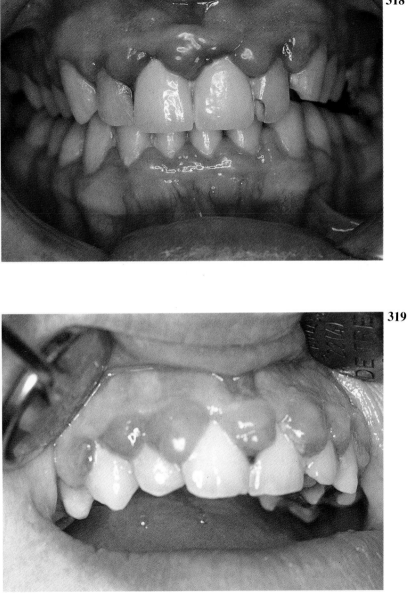

318

319

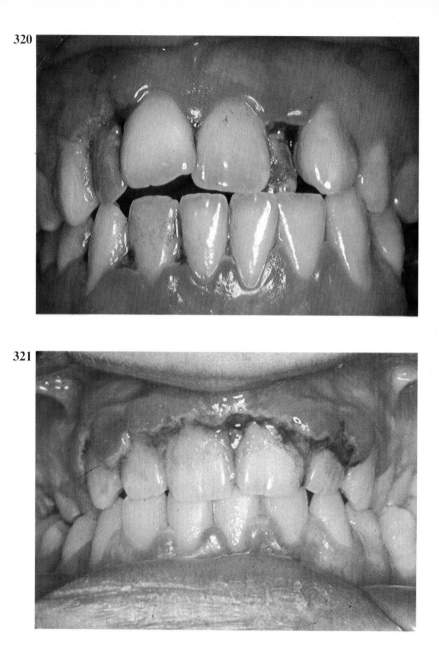

320

321

320,321,322,323,324,325   Acute ulcerative gingivitis   Acute ulcerative gingivitis (Vincent's gingivitis) is by far the most common acute infective condition effectively restricted to the gingivae. Other acute infective gingival conditions (such as herpes simplex, **92**) occur much more commonly as part of a more generalized gingivo-stomatitis. The exact cause of acute ulcerative gingivitis is not known: although invariably associated with the presence of Vincent's organisms (*Borrelia vincenti* and *Fusiformis fusiformis*), it seems that a simple primary infective process is not responsible for the gingivitis. However, there is no doubt that clinical improvement is associated with the elimination of these organisms. These patients illustrate the predominant feature of acute ulcerative gingivitis: the development of crater like ulcers involving the gingival papillae (**320**), followed by lateral spread along the gingival margins (**321,322**). In a few cases, following no treatment

322

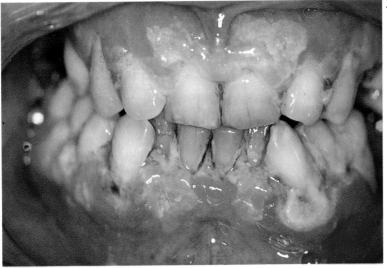

or inadequate treatment, a subacute stage may be reached (**323**). In a very few cases, the condition may be localized to one or a few teeth (**324**). The condition may also, in some few cases, be localized to the area surrounding a partially erupted third molar where stagnation appears to support the conditions necessary for the growth of the organisms (**325**). Generalized ill health may result in either repeated episodes of acute ulcerative gingivitis or, in extreme cases, to rapid and destructive spread of the infection of which cancrum oris (**57**) is the most extreme example.

323

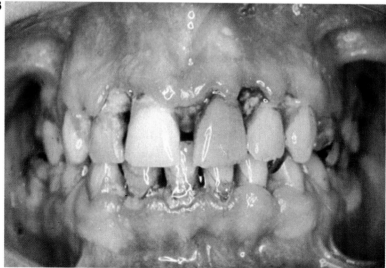

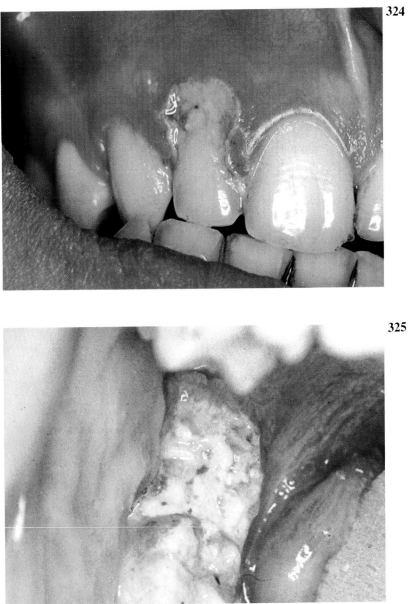

326 Traumatic gingivitis Traumatic gingivitis, caused by over enthusiastic tooth brushing, is not uncommon. There is often some element of an obsessional approach to oral hygiene in patients who present with this condition.

327 Gingivitis artefacta Self inflicted trauma of the gingivae — gingivitis artefacta — is equally not very rare. The patients often profess a great interest in oral hygiene and, to demonstrate, may place their finger nails exactly in the site of such lesions as those seen here.

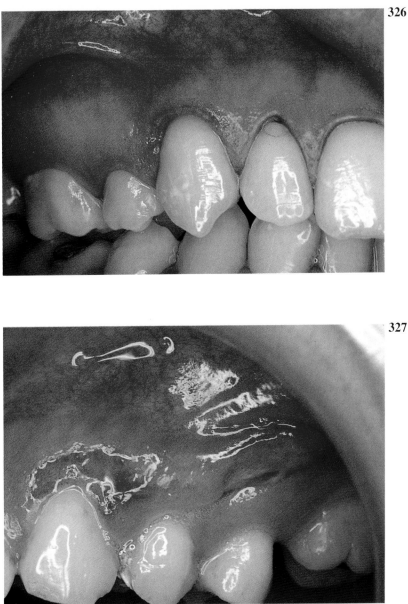

328 Melanotic pigmentation of the gingivae Melanotic pigmentation of the gingivae is common as a normal racial characteristic, as shown here and in **269**. It may also occur much less frequently, together with similar changes elsewhere in the oral mucosa, as a result of drug therapy or of endocrine related disease (**176**).

329 Multiple warts on the gingivae Shown here are multiple warts of the gingivae, associated with others on other sites on the oral mucosa and on the hands. This is a relatively rare presentation, but is almost certainly the result of papillomavirus transmission.

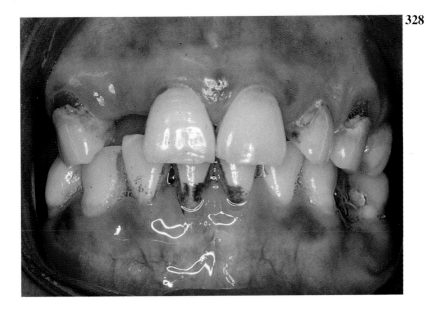

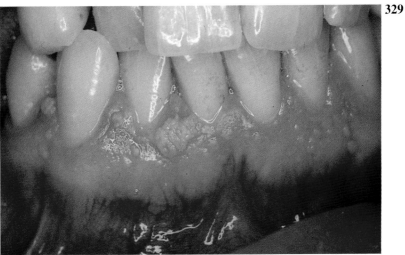

330 Fibro-epithelial polyps on the gingivae These lesions on the gingivae resembled fibro-epithelial polyps rather than papillomas: again, a rare situation but with no known infective, genetic or generalized background in this case.

331 Bismuth line This is a classic, but now virtually never encountered, clinical picture: a bismuth line. This, and the similar lead and mercury lines, were the result of heavy metal deposition in the gingivae. This followed systemic treatment with metal salts for a range of diseases, but usually syphilis.

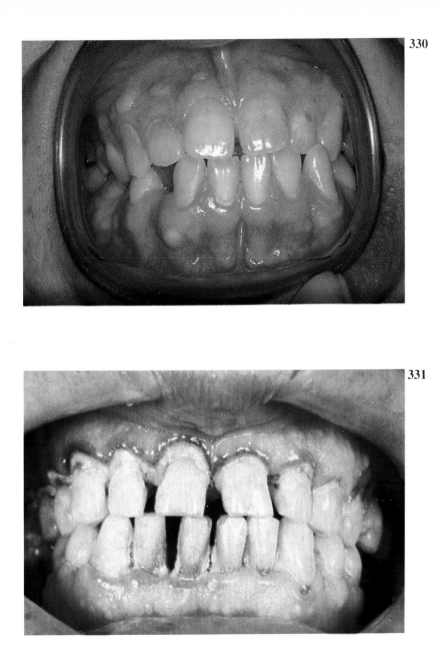

332 Gingival fibromatosis Gingival fibromatosis may exist as a single entity or may also be associated with a wide range of epidermal, skeletal or other defects. In this case there were no other associated features.

333 Large fibrous epulis This is a large fibrous epulis: its structure is not essentially different from the two epulides shown in **334** and **335**, but is more mature, with a predominance of fibrous tissue and a less vascular structure. This demonstrates the size such lesions can attain without causing sufficient problems to force the patient to seek advice.

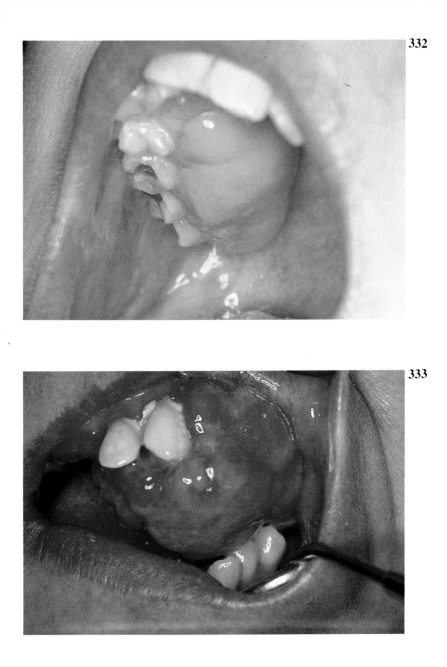

334,335 Epulides Presumably because of the high level of cellular activity, the gingival tissues are particularly susceptible to the production of exuberant inflammatory overgrowths — the epulis series (epulides). These lesions all have the histological appearance of granulation tissue in one or other of its aspects. The lesions shown in **334** and **335** had the histological structure of immature and highly vascular granulation tissue: a structure similar to that of the pregnancy epulis (**317**). The term pyogenic granuloma, often used for lesions such as this, is a historical one in this context and has no good pathological basis.

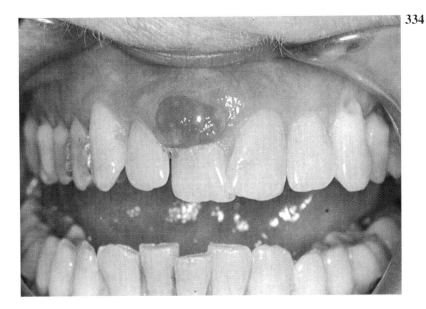

334

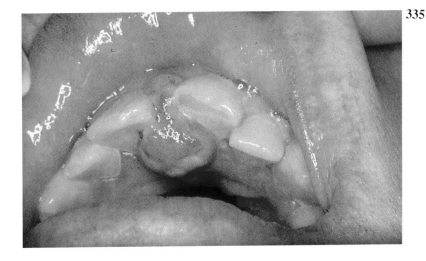

335

336,337   Giant cell epulis   A giant cell epulis such as this (**336**) is differentiated from the simple granulomatous type lesions shown in **333,334** and **335**, by the presence of many osteoclast like giant cells. This is thought to be a reactive lesion, although its exact aetiology is not known. The clinical appearance is generally deep red and often ulcerated. However, some lesions, such as that shown in **337**, are clinically not a great deal different to the non giant cell types. It is important, if such a lesion is diagnosed, to exclude the possibility that the obvious soft tissue swelling is not a peripheral extension of a central giant cell lesion. If a giant cell lesion of the jaws (either central or peripheral) is diagnosed, investigations must be carried out for the possibility of hyperparathyroidism. A giant cell granuloma in an edentulous mouth is shown in **196**.

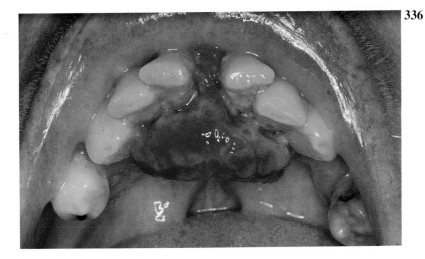

336

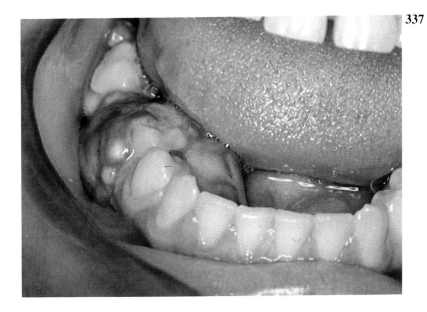

337

275

338 Calcifying epulis This is a calcifying epulis, not very different in its behaviour and structure from a simple fibrous epulis. In fact a calcifying epulis represents only a fibrous epulis that has undergone maturation; some degree of calcification is found in about 30% of all epulides.

339 Lymphoma Malignancy affecting the gingivae in a relatively diffuse manner is very rare. Here, however, is a lymphoma involving the gingival tissues. The description of this in the first edition of this atlas as a reticulum cell sarcoma was in accordance with the then accepted terminology.

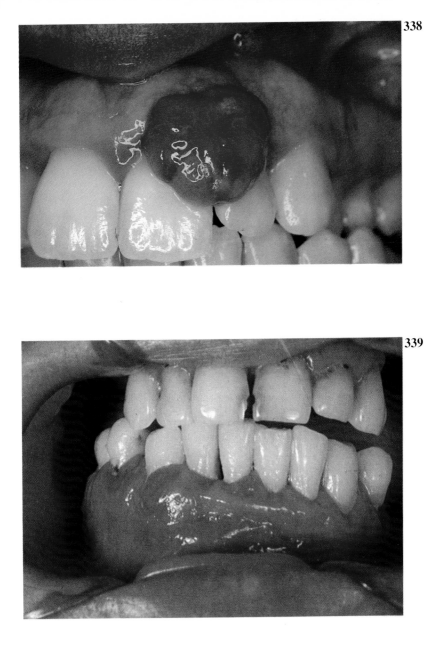

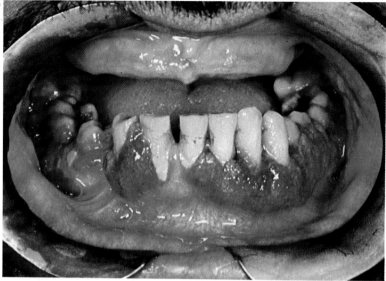

340 Malignant granuloma A quite specific form of gingivitis —
described as having the appearance of raspberries — has been
described in a number of cases of widespread aggressive
granulomatous diseases such as Wegener's granulomatosis and, as in
this case, malignant granuloma of the nasal region. The histology is
non specific and the aetiology of this gingivitis is unknown.

341,342 Histiocytosis X Histiocytosis X is a term used to describe a
group of poorly understood diseases in which various organs are
infiltrated by lesions containing a high proportion of histiocytes and
eosinophils. According to the precise nature of the histology of the
lesions, their distribution in the tissues and the age and other details of
the patient, a range of differing classifications has been suggested by
various authorities. This represents the most common presentation of
such lesions in the jaws: osteolytic lesions apparently centred in or near
the alveolus that leave the affected teeth with virtually no supporting
bone. The localized and apparently relatively minor gingival defect is
characteristic.

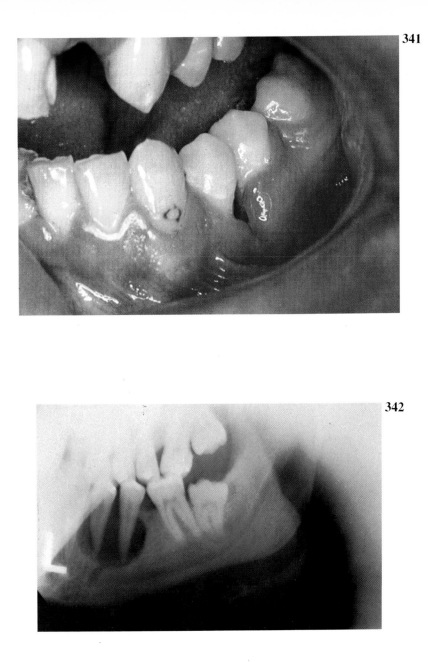

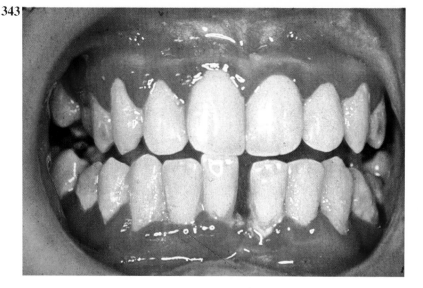

343 Cyclic neutropenia A severe, and often proliferative, gingivitis may occur in leukaemias and also in quantitative disorders of the leukocyte system such as cyclic neutropenia as shown here. In the case of leukaemias the gingivae are found to contain many abnormal leukocytes, whereas in conditions such as cyclic neutropenia the gingival reaction appears to be due to a functional deficiency of the leukocytes, with a resulting disturbance of the protective mechanisms of the gingivae. The picture may be complicated by widespread infective and ulcerative secondary lesions.

Abnormalities of bone

This section includes a number of quite different types of bone disease. The first few examples are of inflammatory and neoplastic bone disorders, others of which have been shown in the section on "Facial swellings".

The later examples are of developmental abnormalities, both of the skull and facial bones as a whole and, particularly from **362** onwards, of disproportionate growth between the skull and jaws that may be susceptible to surgical/orthodontic correction.

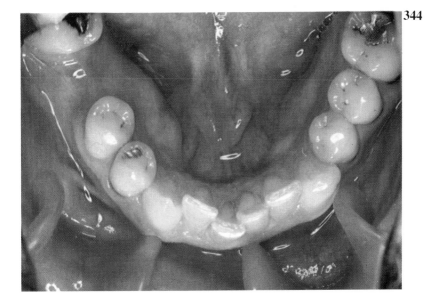

344   Torus mandibularis   These two bony projections on the lingual side of the mandible are static developmental features and very common. This lesion is known as a torus mandibularis. Torus is a term used to describe an outgrowth of bone.

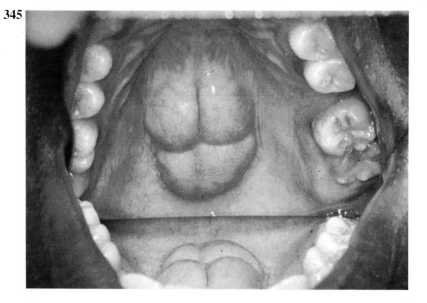

345   Torus palatinus   This is a torus palatinus, the palatal equivalent of the mandibular torus shown in **344**. Like the mandibular torus this is a virtually static and entirely benign lesion, causing problems only when dentures are to be constructed. There may, however, in a few patients be a very slow enlargement measured in years. It must be differentiated from palatal soft tissue swellings, particularly from pleomorphic adenomas such as the one shown in **193**.

346,347   Atrophy of the alveolar bone   These pictures demonstrate a very common problem: that of atrophy of the alveolar bone following tooth loss and the wearing of dentures (flabby ridges). Such alveolar resorption is one of the most frequent causes of difficulty in denture construction.

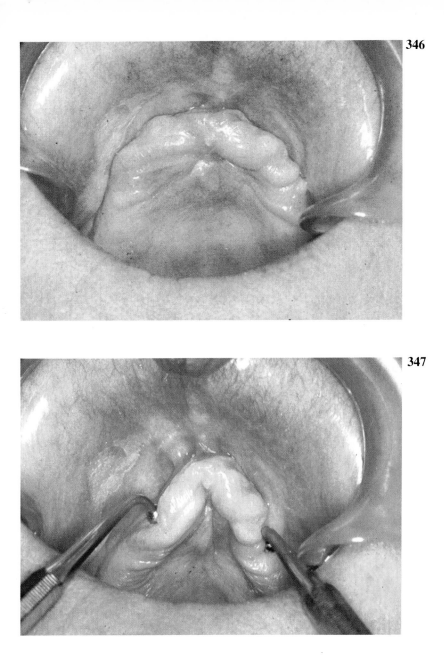

346

347

283

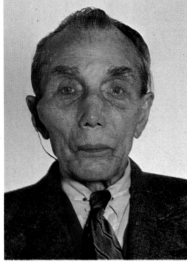

348,349,350 Paget's disease
Paget's disease is a condition of older individuals in which there is an imbalance between the normal processes of bone deposition and resorption. As a result there is overall growth and distortion of the bone. In many cases this is a slow and asymptomatic process: it is found at autopsy in many patients for whom it had not been a clinical problem. In others, however, the bone growth is relatively rapid, leading to distortion of the skull and facial bones (**348**). In particular, there may be growth of the alveolar bone, as shown in **349**. This illustrates also a common complication of Paget's disease — infection and localized osteomyelitis following tooth extraction. The radiograph (**350**) shows the typical thickening of the skull and the cotton wool appearance of the affected bone.

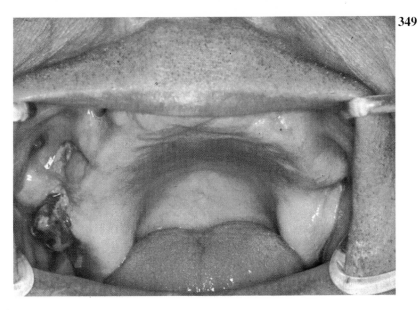

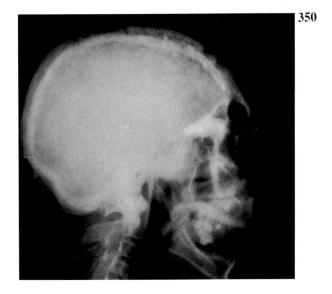

351 Chondroma of the mandible This lesion is an unusual one: a chondroma of the mandible. The symphysis of the mandible is said to be one of the sites at which such lesions most often occur, as are the condylar and coronoid processes. This site distribution is presumably related to the method of growth and development of the mandible. In this case the separation of the teeth as a result of the neoplastic growth is evident. In the mandible, as in other sites, the histological diagnosis of a chondroma, and its differentiation from a chondrosarcoma may be a difficult one. Even with a firm histological diagnosis of a benign neoplasm, the clinical course of any chondrogenic tumour may be more aggressive than expected.

352 Cleft palate A cleft of the secondary palate: only the soft palate is involved. There are many variants. This is included as the simplest example of cleft palate.

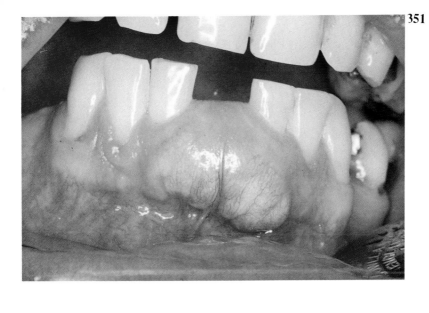

351

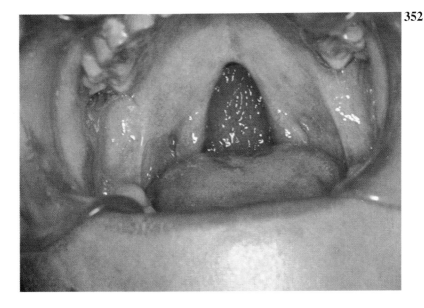

352

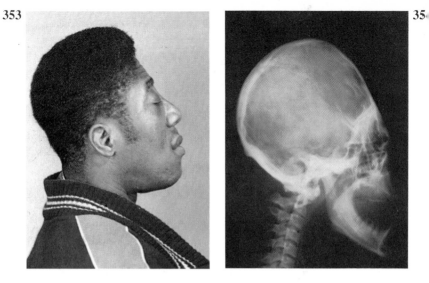

353,354 Oxycephaly There are a range of developmental abnormalities that affect the cranium; this example is oxycephaly. In this condition there is premature closure of the cranial sutures with consequent distortion of the normal skull shape.

355,356,357 Cleidocranial dysostosis Cleidocranial dysostosis is a condition in which there may be failure in development of a number of membrane bones, but particularly the clavicle and the skull. There may also be a number of supernumerary teeth present, often unerupted. **355** shows the characteristic frontal flattening in such a patient. The lack of development of the clavicles is shown in the radiograph **356**. The numerous retained teeth shown in **357** were found in a patient thought to have had all teeth extracted previously. This condition is perhaps the best known of the many in which bones and teeth may be involved in abnormality.

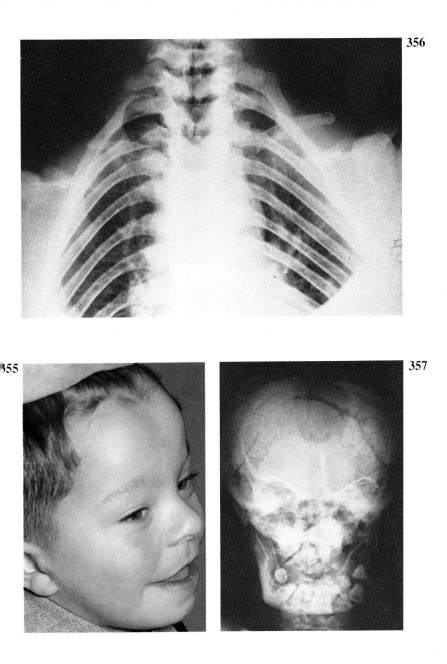

358,359,360,361   First arch syndrome   This is the so called "first arch syndrome". In this condition there is unilateral failure in development of those structures derived from the first branchial arch. The resulting facial asymmetry (due to lack of mandibular development) and malformed ear are shown in **358** and **359**. The consequent dental malocclusion is shown in **360**. The radiograph (**361**) shows the general asymmetry of the facial skeleton.

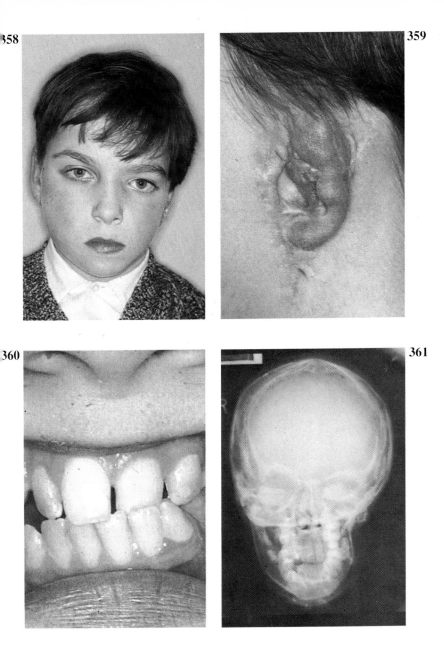

362,363   Anterior open bite   This is an example of anterior open bite in which the abnormality is restricted to the anterior part of the maxillary dentition — the so called "dental" type. The skeletal pattern is otherwise normal as is the posterior occlusion.

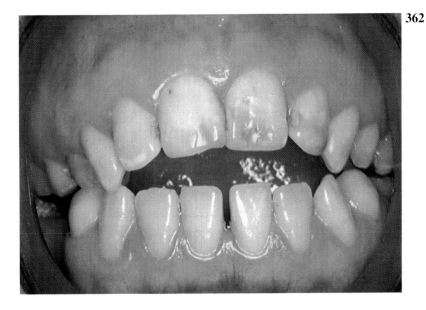

362

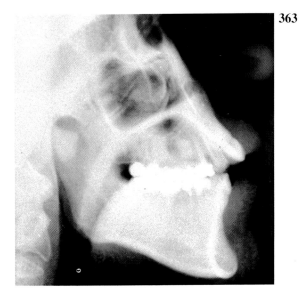

363

364,365 Anterior open bite In contrast to the previous patient, contact here is limited to the second molars, with a progressively increasing discrepancy between the more anterior teeth. This is the "skeletal" pattern of anterior open bite.

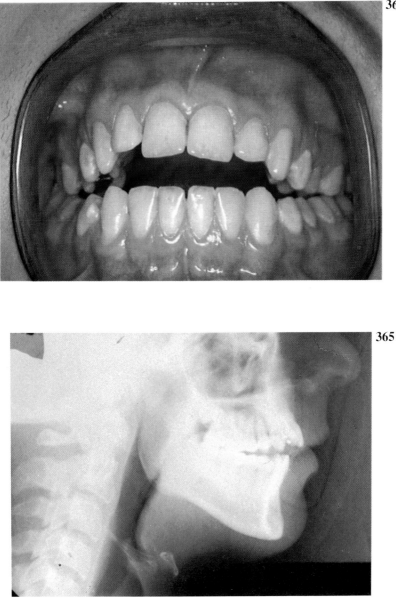

366

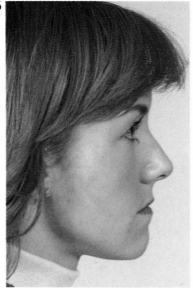

366,367 Mild mandibular prognathism This is an example of mild mandibular prognathism. The resultant dental defect is shown in **367**: the occlusal disharmony has led to temporo-mandibular joint dysfunction symptoms. This problem was dealt with by a push back sagittal split osteotomy (preceded by orthodontic treatment).

367

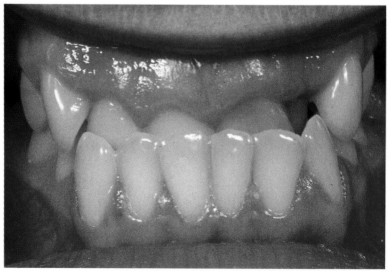

368 Mandibular prognathism
The mandibular prognathism is much more marked in this patient, with an increased mandibular angle and an elongated chin. A patient such as this requires more elaborate treatment than the previous one; in this case a body osteotomy with anterior–posterior and vertical reduction, with genioplasty and maxillary augmentation.

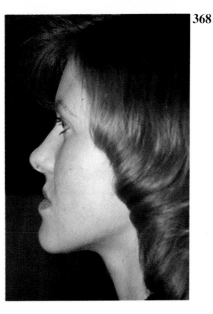

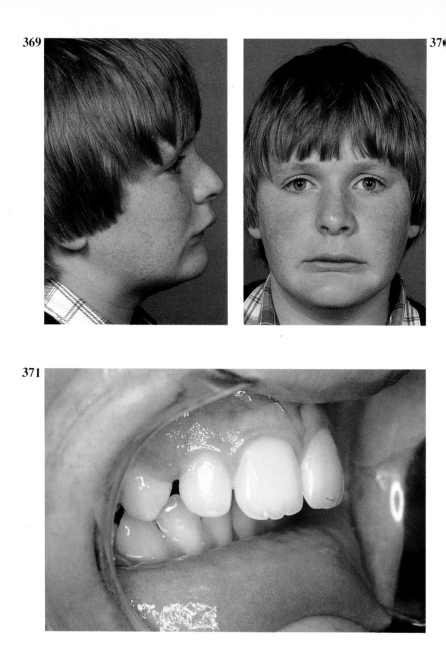

369 370

371

298

369,370,371   Class II malocclusion   This is a patient with a severe Class II skeletally based malocclusion. He had a retrusive mandible with a decreased lower facial height (**370**). There was over eruption of the lower incisors, which were traumatizing the palatal mucosa (**371**). An early mandibular advancement with genioplasty was carried out in this case.

372   Maxillary hypoplasia The essential problem in this case is maxillary hypoplasia and, hence, nasal prominence. Maxillary advancement and rhinoplasty were carried out.

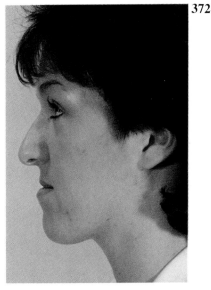

372

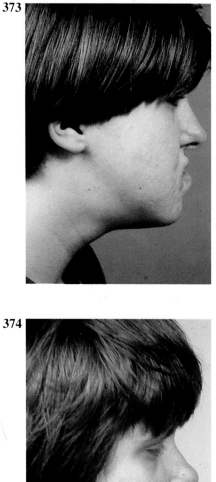

373,374 Maxillary hypoplasia
These are before-and-after pictures of a patient with maxillary hypoplasia following a cleft palate repair in childhood. There was a considerable degree of post cleft hypernasality due to an incompetent velopharyngeal closure. **374** shows the patient after a supra-apical midface osteotomy.

375,376 Maxillary retrusion
This patient appears to have prognathism, but in fact the main problem was maxillary retrusion as a post cleft deformity. This being so, a satisfactory result was obtained by carrying out maxillary surgery without the need for a mandibular osteotomy.

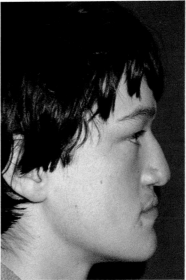

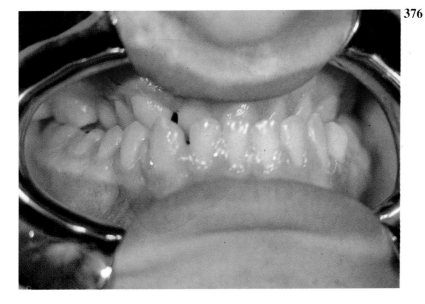

377

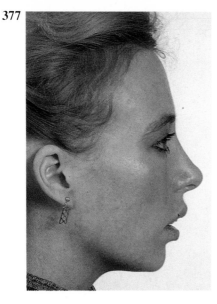

377,378 Vertical maxillary excess An example of lip incompetence resulting from a vertical maxillary excess. The surgery indicated was a reduction of this by a LeFort 1 maxillary osteotomy.

378

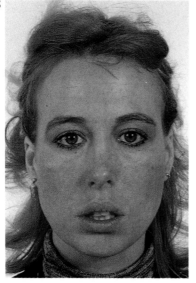

379,380 Mandibular prognathism with maxillary hypoplasia Shown here (**379**) is severe mandibular prognathism associated with maxillary hypoplasia. The results of a bimaxillary osteotomy and genioplasty are shown in **380**.

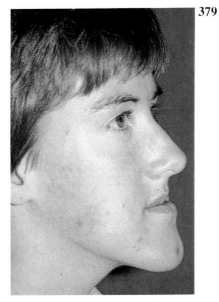

379

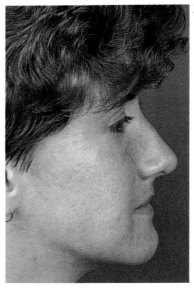

380

381

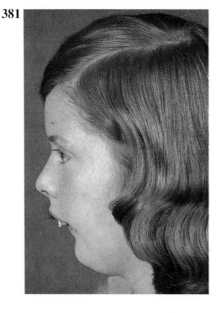

381,382 Severe Class II malocclusion This patient had a severe Class II (division 1) skeletally based malocclusion with a vertical maxillary excess and a retrusive mandible. The lower incisors were occluding in a line drawn between the upper incisors. The angular cheilitis, resulting from the lip incompetence, is evident. The surgical approach was a 3 partate maxillary osteotomy with mandibular advancement.

382

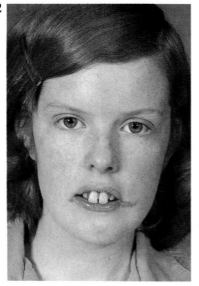

383,384 Vertical maxillary excess A further case of vertical maxillary excess with some deficiency of mandibular growth.

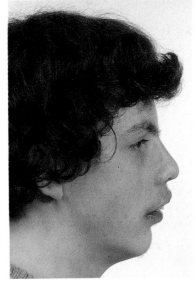

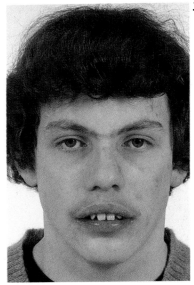

385

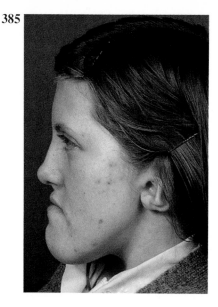

385,386 Klippel–Feil This is the Klippel–Feil syndrome, in which there is midfacial hypoplasia together with true mandibular prognathism. At this age (18 years) the patient had already undergone one operation for maxillary advancement.

386

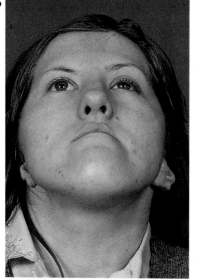

387,388 Post cleft deformity A post cleft deformity, with hypoplasia of the malar/nasal/maxillary complex. The patient had lost his upper teeth at an early stage and the construction of satisfactory dentures was made very difficult by the discrepancy between the arches. Surgical treatment for this included a LeFort II midfacial osteotomy to bring forward the maxilla and malars. This was followed by an augmentation rhinoplasty.

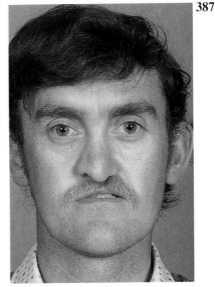

387

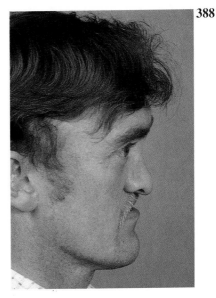

388

389

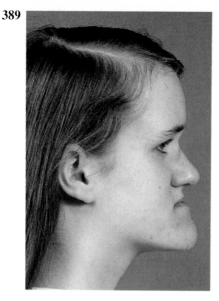

389,390,391 Severe midfacial hypoplasia This patient has severe midfacial hypoplasia that mimics true prognathism. There is also an eccentric position of the chin — not a true mandibular asymmetry. The surgery, therefore, was to the maxilla rather than the mandible: a LeFort III midfacial osteotomy.

390

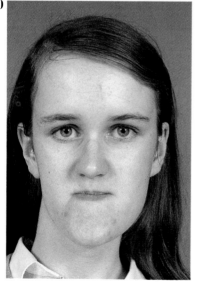

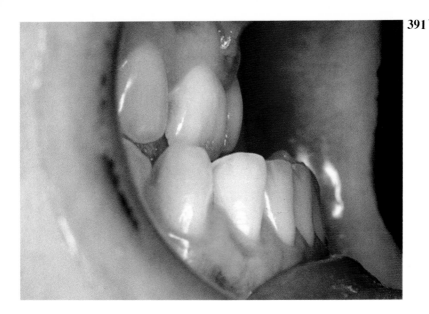

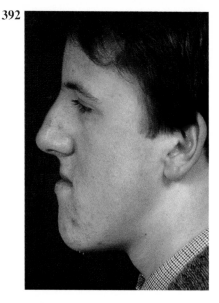

392,393,394 Severe malocclusion The patient shown had a severe malocclusion with contact on two molar teeth only (**394**). He had shortening of the midface but increased dentoalveolar height in the maxilla. He also had mandibular prognathism. In view of the aetiology of the condition, treatment consisted of osteotomies to both the maxilla and the mandible together with a genioplasty.

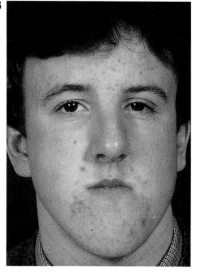

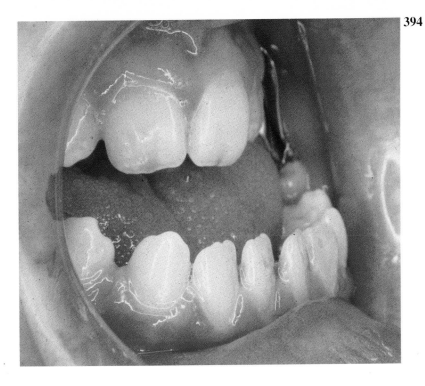

394

Index

References are to figure numbers unless otherwise indicated